Flap Reconstruction of the Traumatized Upper Extremity

Editor

KEVIN C. CHUNG

HAND CLINICS

www.hand.theclinics.com

Consulting Editor
KEVIN C. CHUNG

May 2014 • Volume 30 • Number 2

ELSEVIER

1600 John F. Kennedy Boulevard • Suite 1800 • Philadelphia, Pennsylvania, 19103-2899

http://www.theclinics.com

HAND CLINICS Volume 30, Number 2
May 2014 ISSN 0749-0712, ISBN-13: 978-0-323-29707-3

Editor: Jennifer Flynn-Briggs
Developmental editor: Stephanie Carter

Hand Clinics (ISSN 0749-0712) is published quarterly by Elsevier Inc., 360 Park Avenue South, New York, NY 10010-1710. Months of publication are February, May, August, and November. Business and Editorial Offices: 1600 John F. Kennedy Blvd., Ste. 1800, Philadelphia, PA 19103-2899. Customer Service Office: 3251 Riverport Lane, Maryland Heights, MO 63043. Periodicals postage paid at New York, NY and at additional mailing offices. Subscription price is $390.00 per year (domestic individuals), $606.00 per year (domestic institutions), $194.00 per year (domestic students/residents), $445.00 per year (Canadian individuals), $691.00 per year (Canadian institutions), $530.00 per year (international individuals), $691.00 per year (international institutions), and $256.00 per year (international and Canadian students/residents). Foreign air speed delivery is included in all *Clinics* subscription prices. All prices are subject to change without notice. **POSTMASTER:** Send address changes to *Hand Clinics*, Elsevier Health Sciences Division, Subscription Customer Service, 3251 Riverport Lane, Maryland Heights, MO 63043. Customer Service (orders, claims, online, change of address): Elsevier Health Sciences Division, Subscription Customer Service, 3251 Riverport Lane, Maryland Heights, MO 63043. Tel: 1-800-654-2452 (U.S. and Canada); 314-447-8871 (outside U.S. and Canada). Fax: 314-447-8029. E-mail: journalscustomerservice-usa@elsevier.com (for print support); journalsonlinesupport-usa@elsevier.com (for online support).

Reprints. For copies of 100 or more of articles in this publication, please contact the Commercial Reprints Department, Elsevier Inc., 360 Park Avenue South, New York, New York 10010-1710. Tel.: 212-633-3874; Fax: 212-633-3820; E-mail: reprints@elsevier.com.

Hand Clinics is covered in *MEDLINE/PubMed (Index Medicus), Current Contents/Clinical Medicine, EMBASE/Excerpta Medica,* and *ISI/BIOMED.*

Printed and bound by CPI Group (UK) Ltd, Croydon, CR0 4YY

Contributors

CONSULTING EDITOR

KEVIN C. CHUNG, MD, MS
Charles B.G. de Nancrede Professor of
Surgery, Section of Plastic Surgery,
Department of Surgery; Professor of
Orthopaedic Surgery; Assistant Dean for
Faculty Affairs; Associate Director of Global
REACH, University of Michigan Medical
School, University of Michigan Health System,
Ann Arbor, Michigan

EDITOR

KEVIN C. CHUNG, MD, MS
Charles B.G. de Nancrede Professor of Surgery,
Section of Plastic Surgery, Department of
Surgery; Professor of Orthopaedic Surgery;
Assistant Dean for Faculty Affairs; Associate
Director of Global REACH, University of
Michigan Medical School, University of
Michigan Health System, Ann Arbor, Michigan

AUTHORS

JOSHUA M. ADKINSON, MD
Fellow, Section of Plastic Surgery,
Department of Surgery, University of
Michigan Health System, Ann Arbor,
Michigan

SARAH E. APPLETON, MD, MSc
Plastic and Reconstructive Surgery,
Dalhousie University, Halifax, Nova Scotia,
Canada

BABU BAJANTRI, MS, MCh
Consultant, Department of Plastic
Surgery, Hand and Reconstructive
Microsurgery and Burns, Ganga Hospital,
Coimbatore, India

BRIAN T. CARLSEN, MD
Associate Professor of Plastic Surgery,
College of Medicine, Mayo Clinic,
Rochester, Minnesota

CENK CAYCI, MD
Chief Resident, Division of Plastic and
Reconstructive Surgery; Instructor in Surgery,
College of Medicine, Mayo Clinic, Rochester,
Minnesota

JAMES CHANG, MD
Professor of Surgery and Division Chief,
Division of Plastic and Reconstructive Surgery,
Stanford University Medical Center, Stanford;
Director, Plastic and Hand Surgery Laboratory,
Veterans Affairs Palo Alto Health Care System,
Palo Alto, California

GRACE J. CHIOU, MD
Postdoctoral Research Fellow, Division of
Plastic and Reconstructive Surgery, Stanford
University Medical Center, Stanford;
Postdoctoral Research Fellow, VA Palo Alto
Division of Plastic and Reconstructive Surgery,
Palo Alto, California

KEVIN C. CHUNG, MD, MS
Charles B.G. de Nancrede Professor of
Surgery, Section of Plastic Surgery,
Department of Surgery; Professor of
Orthopaedic Surgery; Assistant Dean for
Faculty Affairs; Associate Director of Global
REACH, University of Michigan Medical
School, University of Michigan Health System,
Ann Arbor, Michigan

FRANK FANG, MD
Chief Resident, Section of Plastic Surgery,
Department of Surgery, The University of
Michigan Health System, Ann Arbor, Michigan

**ANDREW M. HART, BSc, MBChB, MRCS,
AFRCSEd, MD, PhD, FRCSEd (Plast)**
Consultant Plastic Surgeon, Canniesburn
Plastic Surgery Unit, Glasgow Royal Infirmary;
Stephen Forrest Professor of Plastic Surgery,
The University of Glasgow, Glasgow,
United Kingdom

ELIZABETH A. KING, MD
Resident Physician, Department of
Orthopaedic Surgery, University of Michigan,
Ann Arbor, Michigan

STEVEN F. MORRIS, MD, MSc, FRCSC
Professor of Surgery; Professor of Anatomy,
Departments of Surgery, Anatomy and
Neurobiology, Dalhousie University, Halifax,
Nova Scotia, Canada

KAGAN OZER, MD
Associate Professor, Department of
Orthopaedic Surgery, University of Michigan,
Ann Arbor, Michigan

SHADY A. REHIM, MB ChB, MSc, MRCS
International Research Fellow, Section of
Plastic Surgery, Department of Surgery,
University of Michigan Health System,
Ann Arbor, Michigan

**S. RAJA SABAPATHY, MS, MCh, DNB, FRCS
Ed, MAMS**
Chairman, Department of Plastic Surgery,
Hand and Reconstructive Microsurgery and
Burns, Ganga Hospital, Coimbatore, India

MICHEL SAINT-CYR, MD
Professor of Plastic Surgery, College of
Medicine, Mayo Clinic, Rochester, Minnesota

**MARK V. SCHAVERIEN, MBChB, MRCS,
MSc, MEd, MD, FRCSEng (Plast)**
Specialty Registrar in Plastic Surgery,
Department of Plastic and Reconstructive
Surgery, Ninewells Hospital, Dundee,
United Kingdom

**MANEESH SINGHAL, MBBS, MS, MCh,
FACS**
Additional Professor, Department of Surgical
Disciplines, All India Institute of Medical
Sciences (AIMS), New Delhi, India

Contents

An Evolutionary Perspective on the History of Flap Reconstruction in the Upper Extremity   109

Frank Fang and Kevin C. Chung

> Examining the evolution of flap reconstruction of the upper extremity is similar to studying the evolution of biological species. This analogy provides a perspective to appreciate the contributing factors that led to the development of the current arsenal of techniques. It shows the trajectory for the future and provides a glimpse of the factors that that will be influential in the future.

Anatomy and Physiology of Perforator Flaps of the Upper Limb   123

Sarah E. Appleton and Steven F. Morris

> Perforator flaps are an excellent reconstructive option for a functional upper limb reconstruction. This article explores the physiology and general principles of perforator flaps and their indications for use in reconstruction of the upper extremity. Workhorse perforator flaps of the upper extremity, such as the radial artery perforator, ulnar artery perforator, lateral arm perforator, posterior interosseous artery, first dorsal metacarpal artery perforator and perforator-based propeller flaps, are discussed in greater detail.

Local Flaps of the Hand   137

Shady A. Rehim and Kevin C. Chung

> A local flap consists of skin and subcutaneous tissue that is harvested from a site near a given defect while maintaining its intrinsic blood supply. Local skin flaps can be a used as a reliable source of soft tissue replacement that replaces like with like. Flaps are categorized based on composition, method of transfer, flap design, and blood supply, but flap circulation is considered the most critical factor for the flap survival. This article reviews the classification of local skin flaps of the hand and offers a practical reconstructive approach for several soft tissue defects of the hand and digits.

Flap Reconstruction of the Elbow and Forearm: A Case-Based Approach   153

Joshua M. Adkinson and Kevin C. Chung

> Elbow and forearm wounds have distinct reconstructive requirements, but both require a durable and pliable solution. Pedicle, free fasciocutaneous and muscle, and distant (2-stage) flaps have a role in wound reconstruction in these unique areas. This article presents practical surgical cases as a guide to soft tissue reconstruction of the elbow and forearm.

Free Muscle Flaps for Reconstruction of Upper Limb Defects   165

Mark V. Schaverien and Andrew M. Hart

> Restoration of structure, function, and sensation are critical after trauma or tumor resection of the hand. Thorough debridement, reconstruction of functional structures,

and immediate soft tissue coverage are most effectively performed in a single stage within approximately 24 hours of the injury. Skin flaps provide robust, pliable, and cosmetically appropriate tissue that is not prone to contracture and that facilitates secondary reconstructive work. Muscle flaps retain indications for complex defects with substantial initial contamination or dead space, or for reanimation. In this article, the indications, options, and surgical techniques for free muscle flap reconstruction of upper limb defects are reviewed.

Despite the inherent advantages of free flaps for soft tissue cover in upper limb reconstruction, pedicled flaps remain the workhorse in many centers worldwide. Presumed disadvantages of pedicled flaps are that it requires multiple stages, longer hospital stay, are bulky, and primary reconstruction of composite defects cannot be done. Refinements in technique during planning can offset many of the disadvantages. Pedicled flaps are quick and easy to raise and do not need any special microsurgical expertise. Where free flaps are not possible or they fail, pedicled flaps are the lifeboat. An upper limb reconstructive surgeon must be adept at performing these flaps in challenging situations.

Successful soft tissue reconstruction of the upper extremity must provide stable coverage and restore function to the injured hand. To ensure the best possible outcome after traumatic upper extremity injuries, early radical debridement and early flap coverage that restores all missing tissue components is critical to allow early mobilization. Free flaps provide extraordinary versatility in reconstructing defects of soft tissue, muscle, tendon, and bone.

The traumatized hand often has soft tissue loss requiring flap reconstruction. Before proceeding with flap selection, the need for future refinement and secondary surgery should be taken into consideration. Although muscle flaps may offer better contour, fasciocutaneous flaps allow easier secondary flap elevation. After the initial flap reconstruction, indications for secondary procedures may be managed according to tissue type: bone, joint, tendon, nerve, and soft tissue.

This article highlights reconstructive principles in flap selection, use, and insetting to optimize functional and aesthetic outcomes after upper extremity reconstruction. The concept of respecting the aesthetic units of the hand during reconstruction is discussed. A current literature review of the aesthetic outcomes using various flaps, such as fasciocutaneous, fascia only, and muscle flaps, is provided. An approach based on aesthetic unit principles to upper extremity reconstruction is also highlighted to help optimize outcomes.

Dermal Skin Substitutes for Upper Limb Reconstruction: Current Status, Indications, and Contraindications

Shady A. Rehim, Maneesh Singhal, and Kevin C. Chung

Dermal skin substitutes are a group of biologically engineered materials composed of collagen and glycosaminoglycans and are devoid of cellular structures. These biodegradable materials act as an artificial dermis to promote neovascularization and neodermis formation. Their applications in soft tissue reconstructions are rapidly expanding. In this article, the indications, advantages, and limitations of dermal skin substitutes for reconstruction of soft tissue defects of the upper extremity are reviewed.

HAND CLINICS

Preface

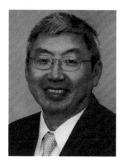

Kevin C. Chung, MD, MS
Editor

A major advance in hand surgery is the understanding of the angiosome concept in which a vessel supplies a distinct area of the skin territory to provide elegant flap coverage for traumatic or chronic wounds. Hand surgeons have become adept anatomists, capable of defining the interplay between vessels and the blood supply of muscle and skin. In recent years, more vascular anatomy has been discovered to identify perforating vessels from major arteries to solve complex wound problems using these so-called perforator vessels. This issue updates the readership regarding the traditional approach for coverage of upper extremity wounds and new solutions using these novel flap techniques.

This issue of *Hand Clinics* is a comprehensive presentation of all the possibilities for wound coverage of the upper extremity and also includes a historical perspective on the evolution of flap procedures that have made salvage of the upper limb a routine practice. Contributions from pioneers in various continents have provided unique solutions that are not constrained by the reconstructive ladder by moving from the simplest techniques such as skin grafting to complex free-flap coverage. In some situations, the most difficult free-style flap option in which an un-named perforator is identified to design a skin paddle provides the best aesthetic appearance after reconstruction. Flap surgery of the upper limb has evolved from simply "stuffing" the hole with bulky muscle flaps to much more selective

choices of distinct flaps that replace like with like using respected anatomic subunits of the hand and upper limb. This provides better function and more aesthetically appealing coverage.

I am grateful to the contributing authors, who shared their insight by providing practical advice on various options for a multitude of wound situations in the upper limb. All the articles emphasize clarity of concept and describe procedures that are safe and predictable. I hope that this issue can give the readers an up-to-date understanding of flap options when faced with difficult situations that require a creative solution. As Editor of *Hand Clinics*, I am grateful to Jennifer Flynn-Briggs, who has entrusted me to provide descriptions of cutting-edge discoveries in hand surgery in areas that are germane to current practice. I am grateful to the readers for their interest and support of this important journal. I am looking forward to your advice on topics that interest you and can be helpful to your practices.

Sincerely,

Kevin C. Chung, MD, MS
Section of Plastic Surgery, Department of Surgery
University of Michigan Medical School
Ann Arbor, MI 48109, USA

E-mail address:
kecchung@med.umich.edu

http://dx.doi.org/10.1016/j.hcl.2013.12.002
0749-0712/14/$ – see front matter

An Evolutionary Perspective on the History of Flap Reconstruction in the Upper Extremity

Frank Fang, MD, Kevin C. Chung, MD, MS*

KEYWORDS

• Upper extremity • Flap reconstruction • History

KEY POINTS

- The evolution of flap reconstruction of the upper extremity can be summarized in the format of a phylogenetic tree.
- The history of upper extremity flap reconstruction can be organized into 5 major eras.
- In the nineteenth and early twentieth centuries, progress in upper extremity flap reconstruction followed the breakthroughs in head and neck reconstruction.
- From the 1990s to the present time, flap reconstructive techniques have been developed that are unique to the upper extremity.

INTRODUCTION

Studying the development of flap reconstructive modalities of the upper extremity is similar to tracking the evolution of a species from its precursors. Similar to how a species evolves a niche because of environmental factors and resources that are present, the techniques of upper extremity flap reconstruction have developed primarily in response to 3 factors: trauma generated by the maiming insults of war and industry, knowledge exchange, and technology. This article presents this story from an evolutionary perspective that guides the reader through the development of each class of upper extremity flap reconstruction from the roots in ancient time to the distal branches of recent time. Readers should note the consistent theme of derivation from head and neck reconstructive methods that characterizes the early years of upper extremity flap reconstruction. This story organizes into 5 eras of time (**Fig. 1**). The period from antiquity to the Industrial Revolution (~1760–1820) is notable for bringing core anatomic knowledge, early principles of plastic surgery, and improvements in trauma care. The next time period spans the 1800s through the end of World War I and is most notable for key scientific breakthroughs and the propagation of plastic surgery. The following time period that is discussed is the interwar period through the end of World War II. The first Great War had generated a huge reconstructive case volume that catalyzed the maturation of plastic surgical reconstruction of the head and neck. The first applications of these plastic surgical principles to the hand after World War I marked the arrival of a new specialty: hand

Funding Sources: Frank Fang, nil; Kevin C. Chung, research reported in this publication was supported by the National Institute of Arthritis and Musculoskeletal and Skin Diseases of the National Institutes of Health under award number K24 AR053120.
Conflict of Interest: None.
Section of Plastic Surgery, Department of Surgery, The University of Michigan Health System, 2130 Taubman Center, SPC 5340, 1500 East Medical Center Drive, Ann Arbor, MI 48109-5340, USA
* Corresponding author.
E-mail address: kecchung@med.umich.edu

Hand Clin 30 (2014) 109–122
http://dx.doi.org/10.1016/j.hcl.2013.12.001
0749-0712/14/$ – see front matter © 2014 Elsevier Inc. All rights reserved.

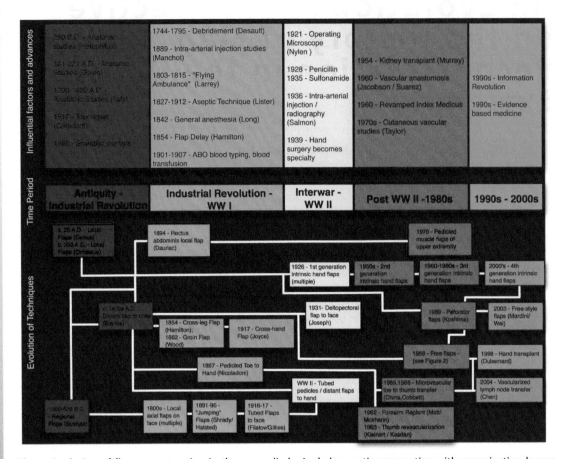

Fig. 1. Evolution of flap reconstruction in the upper limb. A phylogenetic perspective with organization by era and influential factors.

surgery. The next time period, the post–World War II era, is most notable for trauma from modern tools. This time period continues with an evolution upper extremity flap reconstruction that lags slightly behind that of head and neck reconstruction. Microvascular surgery also arrives during this era. It is not until the fifth time period (1990s–2010s) when flap reconstruction in the upper extremity takes a unique course of development by combining reconstructive principles in a way not yet seen before on other parts of the body. This most recent time is also notable for the impact of evidence-based medicine in guiding the implementation of techniques that are available.

ANTIQUITY TO THE INDUSTRIAL REVOLUTION
Early Antiquity: Accumulation of Core Anatomic Knowledge and the Initial Principles of Plastic Surgery

The evolution of the specialty of plastic surgery and basis for upper extremity flap reconstruction

begins in antiquity. Early Indian and Greek cultures showed enormous potential for advancing plastic surgery. Susruta of India (~1000–800 BC) described a regional pedicled flap for the nose in *Samahita*. Significant anatomic discoveries occurred in ancient Greek and Roman civilizations. Herophilus of Chalcedon (c. 250 BC) performed the first scientifically documented human cadaver dissections in Alexandria, Egypt (the only academic arena in ancient Greece where cadaver dissections were legal). Galen (131–221 AD) of the subsequent Roman culture described muscular anatomy from a perspective that was based on both his interpretation of Herophilus' records and also his dissections of animals. During Roman times, Celsus (25 AD) and Oribasius (325–403 AD) described random circulation pedicled flaps and local tissue rearrangements for the lips, nose, ears, and forehead. This era had all of the critical factors that would drive the accelerated course of evolution of upper extremity flap reconstruction seen during the early twentieth century (anatomic investigation, surgical technique innovations, and trauma from war). However, because of the language and communication barriers of this time period, the early techniques of plastic surgery during Indian and Greek cultures developed in parallel and never combined to yield an even greater advancement. The collapse of the Roman Empire ushered in the Dark Ages of Europe. This period of time is marked by frequent warfare and a virtual disappearance of urban life, bringing plastic surgery development to a standstill. Henceforth, no similar skin flap work was recorded for many centuries.

Antiquity (After the Dark Age): Rediscovery and Progress in Anatomy and Plastic Surgical Technique

The early medieval period of Europe is marked by retracing and building on the discoveries of early antiquity. Anatomic discovery, which had remained stagnant from the time of Galen's reports until exploration resumed in the twelfth to thirteenth centuries, resumed with the University of Bologna (Italy) group of anatomists. Ugo Borgognoni of Lucca and his son Theodoric of Cervia conducted human cadaver dissections on executed criminals. This practice was acceptable at the University of Bologna because it was not affiliated with the Catholic Church. Guglielmo da Saliceto (1210–1277 AD) described motor nerves for the first time. Mondino de Liuzzi (1270–1326 AD) was the first anatomist to inject colored liquids into blood vessels, a method that made study of the circulatory system possible; investigators used variants of this technique in the nineteenth and twentieth centuries to define the vascular supply of flaps elevated for reconstructive surgery. In the 1400s, European surgeons rediscovered the flap techniques of ancient India. Gustavo Branca of Italy began using the locoregional forehead flap technique of Susruta for the nose. There is speculation that the original Indian texts of Susruta had been translated to Arabic, which ultimately traveled to Italy and the Brancas. This development marked what was likely the first international exchange of technical knowledge; one of the major factors affecting the evolution of upper extremity flap reconstruction. The exact details and dates are uncertain because the Brancas were very secretive.[1] Gustavo Branca's son Antonio began using a distant flap reconstruction for the nose as harvested from the arm, which is the first documented use of the upper extremity as a donor site for flap reconstruction. The Vianeo brothers of Calabria and Heinrich von Pfolsprundt (c. 1450) of Germany also used this technique for distant flap reconstruction of the nose. Gaspare Tagliacozzi (1545–1599), a professor of anatomy and surgery

at the University of Bologna, finally published the technique with hopes of distributing it widely. However, the surgical community of that era did not embrace his technique, and the use of skin flaps died away again in the Western world. However, despite another stagnation in evolution of plastic surgical technique, anatomic knowledge relevant to flap reconstruction advanced steadily. The use of the printing press during the fifteenth to sixteenth centuries allowed wide distribution of this knowledge. Upper extremity anatomic depictions made significant advances in accuracy with the work of the Renaissance scientist-artists Michelangelo Buonarroti (1475–1564) and Leonardo da Vinci (1452–1519). Berengario da Carpi (1460–1530) of the University of Bologna produced detailed depictions of both the abdominal musculature and upper extremity vasculature. Giovanni Battista Canano of Ferrara (1515–1579) produced excellent illustrations of muscles of the upper extremity in his *Muscolorum Humani Corporis Picturata Dissectio.*[2] During this period, the Belgian anatomist Andreas Vesalius working in Padua published *Humana Corporis Fabrica* (1543), the accuracy and detail of which led him to become known as the reformer of anatomy. Shortly thereafter, Charles Estienne's publication of *De Dissectione Portium Corporis* was released in 1545, which included the first descriptions of superficial nervous and vascular systems. At around the same time, Eustachius of Rome in 1552 was producing anatomic depictions that medical historians contend are even more accurate than, and just as important as, Vesalius' contributions, but these studies were less immediately impactful because of the delay in their publication until 1714.[3] The British great William Harvey delineated the concept of arterial inflow and venous outflow in the extremities with his tourniquet experiment on the forearm and hand in his 1628 book *An Anatomical Study of the Motion of the Heart and of the Blood in Animals*. This period of time in the fifteenth and sixteenth centuries constituted the greatest leap forward of anatomic knowledge in history. This anatomic foundation was the basis for the development of flap reconstructive technique.

Limb Injuries in Antiquity

Before the Industrial Revolution, major extremity injuries with significant soft tissue damage occurred most commonly during war. Gunshot injuries accounted for a growing proportion of battle wounds from the 1400s onward. Because of ineffective hemorrhage control and inadequate measures to prevent and treat infection, major extremity injuries frequently led to death by either initial exsanguination or eventual sepsis. The fundamental principles of military trauma care and lifesaving technology had to develop before extremity reconstruction became a priority. The ancient Chinese, Greeks, and Arabs (900–1000 AD) were the first to try to treat war injuries by such measures as thermal cautery and ephedra-impregnated dressings.[4–6] Extremity trauma surgery during the late medieval period (1500s) only advanced as far as applying ligatures for directed hemostasis and stopping the destructive practice of treating contamination by pouring boiling hot oil on wounds.[3,5] Prussian Hans von Gersdorff first used tourniquetlike devices for amputations in 1517,[7–9] but at that stage extremity salvage was not a realistic goal in trauma triage and management.

INDUSTRIAL REVOLUTION TO WORLD WAR I
The 1700s to 1800s: the Industrial Revolution

The technologic advances of the Industrial Revolution in the 1770s promoted the evolution of flap reconstruction in many ways. Mechanization proved to be equally destructive to the inadvertently placed extremity as it was productive in bringing forth industrial and agricultural output.[10] These extremity injuries provided case volume for extremity reconstruction. The industrial era also brought a large-scale production of war machinery that encouraged widespread use of more destructive weapons than before, and creating more extremity trauma to reconstruct. In addition to additional trauma volume for reconstruction, the Industrial Revolution marked the beginning of a more accelerated pace for dissemination of medical knowledge. With higher output printing presses now available, medical journals arrived in the 1660s and propagated technical and conceptual breakthroughs more efficiently than in any previous era. This technologic advance manifested with the increasingly common use of references to volumes of surgical literature and books by surgeons describing new techniques.[10,11]

Developments in Surgery

This era of surgery is notable for important advances that prepared the way for the major reconstructive extremity surgeries that arrived later in the century. Eighteenth century extremity surgery is notable for the first description of a definitive debridement by Pierre Joseph Desault (1789), a French surgeon of the Napoleonic era.[12] However, this sound surgical technique for trauma inexplicably fell out of favor. As recently as the American Civil War, when 70% of traumatic injuries involved the limbs, excisional debridement was performed in as few as 3% of traumatic wounds. Amputation was the greatly favored treatment option, accounting for approximately 75% of surgeries performed during the American Civil War.[13,14] It was not until World War I when debridement regained acceptance by the influence of the Belgian Antoine Depage.[12] Dominique Jean Larrey introduced effective trauma triage with his so-called flying ambulance during the Napoleonic Wars (1803–1815). This method addressed major trauma with highly efficient mobile medical units close to the lines of battle. The general anesthetic revolution brought about by Crawford Long (1842) and later William G. Morton (1846) was an absolute prerequisite for the lengthy reconstructive surgeries that would evolve in the twentieth century.[3] Aseptic technique with carbolic acid and calcium chlorate described by The United Kingdom's Sir Joseph Lister (1867) and Hungary's Ignaz Philip Semmelweis (1847), along with sulfonamide antibiotics that became widely available in 1938,[15] dramatically reduced infection rates and increased survival from trauma. ABO blood typing, discovered in 1901, yielded the lifesaving tool of blood transfusion in 1907.[16] It was by these technologic breakthroughs and advances of trauma care that soldiers began to survive major trauma with higher frequency.[17] By the start of World War II, mortality for those wounded had decreased to 4.5% from 15% in the American Civil War,[5] and surgeons at last had the option of pursuing limb salvage.[18]

Facial Reconstruction Establishes the Principles of Flap Reconstruction of the Upper Extremity

In addition to trauma caused by war, the late 1700s and 1800s are notable for an influx of facial soft tissue defects created by new extirpative approaches for treating skin cancer. This development spurred a new burst of evolution of flap reconstructive concepts that were later applied to the upper extremity. Francois Chopart of France (1743–1795) began performing advancement flaps for lip reconstruction. Joseph C. Carpue (1764–1846) reintroduced the Indian forehead flap technique that he had learned from reports from surgeons who had traveled to India.[3] Surgeons such as Johann Carl Georg Fricke, Léon Tripier, Karl August von Burow, Jakob August Estlander, Robert Abbe, and Johann Friedrich Dieffenbach began using the readily available axial circulation available in the well-vascularized tissue of the face with various local and regional flaps. Their names have since become eponymous with local flaps on the face. Shrady[19] and Halsted[20] also introduced the walking or jumping flaps for facial reconstruction in the 1890s.

Flap Reconstruction Reaches the Extremities and Trunk

Availability of medical literature now allowed the established reconstructive methods for the face to drive the subsequent evolution of reconstruction on the extremities and trunk. In 1854, years after the first distant flap to the face, Hamilton[21] performed the first distant flap to an extremity with his cross-leg flap, treating a chronic ulcer in a 15-year-old boy with clear reference to "plastic operations" of the past.[22] Hamilton[21] also recognized and described the benefits of flap delay.[21,23] Shortly thereafter, in 1862, Wood[24] described, with clear reference to the "Tagliacotian principle," the first distant flap coverage for upper extremity defects with his axial-patterned circulation groin flap for reconstruction of a cicatricial burn scar contracture on the upper extremity of an 8-year-old girl. However, this technique did not become popular until a half-century later.[24,25] Muscle flaps originated in 1894 with Dauriac of France and with Wolkowicz of Poland in 1895, applying the pedicled transposition concept of the face to the rectus abdominis muscle for reconstruction of abdominal hernias. Shortly thereafter, Tansini[26] and Ombredanne[27] described pedicled muscle flap transpositions of the latissimus dorsi in 1896 and pectoralis major in 1906 respectively for reconstruction of chest wall defects from breast cancer. In 1897, Carl Nicoladoni applied the distant flap concept with a pedicled thoracoepigastric flap to cover a degloved thumb.[28,29] Nicoladoni later further developed the distant flap concept with application to finger reconstruction in his description of a pedicled second toe to thumb transfer in 1900.[29] In 1917, another distant flap for finger reconstruction, the cross-hand flap (substitution of ring finger for reconstruction of a thumb) was performed by J. Leonard Joyce.[30,31] Later, in 1919, Albee[32] developed an osteoplastic finger substitute that combined a bone graft with a distant flap. Albee[32] also clearly indicates the source of inspiration for his technique is the "Italian plastic method."[32] It is notable that Nicoladoni had proposed Albee's reconstructive strategy years earlier, although he had never performed it.

World War I

From the perspective of upper extremity flap reconstruction, World War I was important for 2 reasons. First, it established principles of soft tissue reconstruction on the head and neck that were later used on the upper extremity. Second, the consequences of the unreconstructed upper extremities of this war convinced the medical community that hand surgery was a necessary specialty. Contributions came from Johannes Frederick Esser, Harold Gillies, Varaztad H. Kazanjian, John Staige Davis, Vilray Blair, and Robert H. Ivy, who made significant progress in the reconstruction of disfigured faces by testing and optimizing the reconstructive principles of the nineteenth century surgeons.[33] Tubed pedicled flaps were also introduced during this period by Vladmir Petrovich Filatov in 1916 and Harold Gillies in 1917. The tubed technique provided easier maintenance and better viability for distant flaps. World War I served as the proving ground and engine for propagation of the principles of plastic surgery. As Davis[34] stated, "at the beginning of World War I, there were, with the exception of myself, no general plastic surgeons available in the U.S." By the time of the start of World War II, there were at least 60 practicing plastic surgeons in the United States.[35] World War I was characterized by a lack of treatment of hand injuries,[36,37] as shown by only a half dozen scattered references to hand injuries from the surgical volumes documenting World War I in contrast with the 419-page volume on hand surgery produced after World War II by Bunnell.[36,37]

WORLD WAR I TO WORLD WAR II
Interwar Period

After World War I, surgeons realized the impact of the disability caused by a major upper extremity injury. In assessing the injuries from World War I, Surgeon General Norman T. Kirk and the so-called father of hand surgery Dr Sterling Bunnell stated, "a man without a functional hand was the equivalent of a man without a hand." By their influence, there was now a growing appreciation for the magnitude of the disabling effect of a crippled hand on an individual and the criteria by which specific hand disabilities would disqualify an individual from military service.[36] Thus, there was now a commitment to addressing major upper extremity trauma that would be notably present during World War II.[35]

In the meantime, hand trauma caused by the new age of electric machines and tools of industrial work during the interwar period drove the evolution of a first generation of intrinsic hand flaps; techniques of reconstruction that reside within the limited surface area of the hand (**Fig. 2**).[38] These first intrinsic flaps used the major concepts of plastic surgery established thus far: distant flaps, advancement flaps, and transposition flaps. Gatewood[39] introduced the first distant flap of the

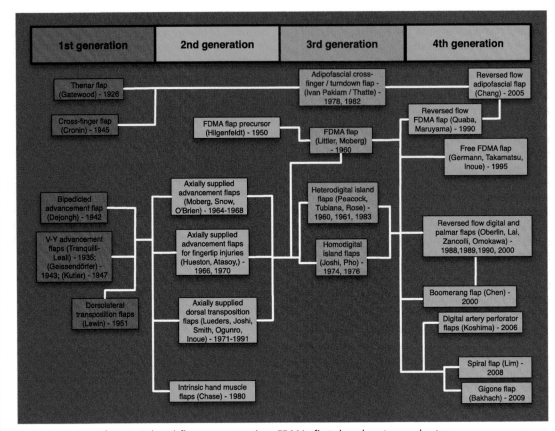

Fig. 2. Evolution of intrinsic hand flap reconstruction. FDMA, first dorsal metacarpal artery.

hand in 1926 with the thenar flap for index fingertip reconstruction. Advancement and transposition flaps were performed in 1935 by Ettore Tranquilli Leali, an Italian surgeon who described the use of the V-Y advancement flap on the volar fingertip, which would become modified and popularized in later years as the Atasoy flap, an axially supplied version of the V-Y advancement.

World War II

The World War II era is notable for the impact of war injuries, industrial trauma, and dissemination of medical literature on the evolution of upper extremity flap reconstruction. Battle injuries from World War II presenting to the hand surgeons of this era, including Sterling Bunnell, Archibald McIndoe, Guy Pulvertaft, Harvey Allen, Ather Cleveland, Eugene Bricker, Don Pratt, Samuel B. Fowler, Major Joseph H. Boyes, Robert L. Payne, and Darrel T. Shaw, required reconstructions using the tubed pedicle flaps and distant flaps (hypogastric-groin flap[40] and thoracoepigastric flaps) learned from head and neck reconstruction in World War I. The expansion of manufacturing labor in World War II also generated an influx of

associated hand trauma, catalyzing further evolution of the first generation of intrinsic hand flaps. Edwin DeJongh[41] described bipedicled advancements for volar fingertip coverage in 1942 for factory-related injuries. H. Geissendörfer of Germany, with his lateral V-Y fingertip advancement in 1943, and William Kutler of the United States with bipedicled lateral V-Y advancement flaps, were inspired by the work of Tranquili-Leali.[42,43] As medical literature became more accessible, the clear evidence of the influence of previous work became present in the cited bibliographies.

AFTER WORLD WAR II

From the standpoint of upper extremity flap reconstruction, the post–World War II period is notable for persistent evolutionary pressure from electric devices causing trauma to the hands. Access to previously published literature also facilitates rediscovery of past techniques. This era witnessed a maturation of medical technologies and techniques leading to the breakthrough technique of microvascular free tissue transfer. This time period marks the beginning of an information revolution in health care. Catalogs of archived literature provide a more accessible resource for exploring the knowledge of the past to fuel future progress.

Additional First-generation Intrinsic Hand Flaps

The increased potential for finger trauma created by the threat of machinery was shown by the spike in patents for safety measures such as guards to be built into saws and other potentially damaging machines.[44] As noted surgeon of this era Edwin DeJongh[41] stated, "In America's large industrial plants, amputation is approaching a rarity. In the smaller jobbing shops, where safety departments are less efficient, this injury is still sadly common." To treat these injuries, surgeons devised additional first-generation intrinsic hand flaps (see **Fig. 2**). Gudin and Pangman[45] reported the distant flap of the hand (the cross-finger flap) in 1950, but it was Cronin[46] who first performed these flaps in 1945 to treat injuries during World War II. The dorsolateral transposition flaps on the fingers, described by Lewin[47] in 1951, harnessed random-patterned blood supply, a concept that had been established on the face in previous years. Again, there is the effect of an increasingly accessible medical literature with techniques that were reported years earlier becoming rediscovered and popularized during this period of time. For instance, the previously reported thenar flap of Gatewood[39] was popularized by Flatt[48] in 1955.

Second-generation Intrinsic Hand Flaps

The persistent demand for finger reconstruction during the postwar period drove the evolution of a second generation of intrinsic hand flaps that are characterized by axially patterned blood supply. This evolution of use of axial blood supply follows the same course that had occurred in flap reconstruction of the face years earlier. The precursor to the first dorsal metacarpal artery (FDMA) flap was described by the German Hilgenfeldt[49] in 1950. However, because of the inaccessibility of the literature generated by Hilgenfeldt,[49] this flap was developed in parallel by J. William Littler and Erik Moberg's description in 1960.[50,51] J. Holevich, Guy Foucher, and Jean-Bernard Braun modified the technique in later years into the present form of the axial-patterned FDMA flap. The analogous flag flap designed for the other fingers was reported by the French hand surgeon Vilain[52] in 1952. It relies on an axial-pattern blood supply to allow the flap to avoid the constraint of the length/width ratio of a standard random-pattern cross-finger flap.[52] The flag flap was further refined by Iselin[53] and eventually Lister.[54] John Wesley Snow, Bernard O'Brien, and Erik

Moberg developed axial-pattern advancement flaps to cover even greater surface areas of fingertip or thumb tip amputations.[55–57] Other surgeons, such as Harold Lueders, Brij Bhushan Joshi, P.J. Smith, Olayinka Ogunro, and Goro Inoue,[58–62] modified the design of the dorsal transposition of Lewin[47] to take advantage of anatomic studies of the axial-patterned blood supply as clarified by Flint and Harrison,[63] Levame and colleagues,[64] and Flint.[65] Hueston[66] and Atasoy and colleagues[67] also reported a similar axially supplied rotational solution to fingertip amputations. The second-generation flaps generally provided more robust coverage with a greater distance of potential advancement and rotation than the previous first-generation flaps.

Head and Neck Concepts Translated to the Upper Extremity

The aforementioned factors of industrial trauma and accessibility of medical literature also spurred the evolution of previously established head and neck reconstructive techniques into their upper extremity forms. In 1957, McCash,[68] and Von Deilen and Coxau[69] formally described the cross-arm flap, although these investigators acknowledged that this technique had likely been used for years by plastic surgeons without ever being specifically reported in the literature. McGregor and Jackson[70] also translated the deltopectoral flap of Vahram Bakamjian and Jacques Joseph into the realm of hand reconstruction in 1970.

Free Flaps Arrive

During the 1960s, advances in several different areas combined to manifest with the arrival of free microvascular tissue transfer (**Fig. 3**). Julius Jacobson and Ernesto Suarez perfected vascular anastomotic technique on dogs and rabbits by 1960. To perform these anastomoses, they had modified the operating microscope from the Zeiss-Littman version that was being used for auricular surgery.[71] Next, Malt and McKhann[72] performed the first successful replantation of a forearm in 1962. Using loupe magnification, Morton Kasdan and Harold Kleinert revascularized an amputated thumb in 1963.[73,74] Yoshio Nakayama and colleagues then completed the first free flap transfer of segments of intestine to the head and neck region in 1964. Surgeons in China performed the first extremity free flap of a microvascular toe to thumb transfer in 1965, but their work remained unknown to the rest of the world until years later because of the political isolation of that time.[75,76] In 1968, The United Kingdom's Cobbett[77] performed the first publicized toe to

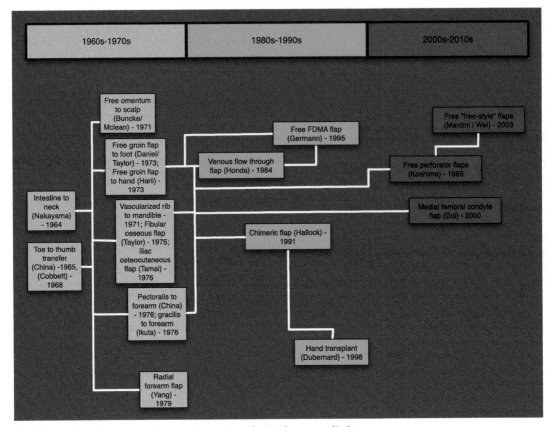

Fig. 3. Evolution of microvascular free tissue transfer in the upper limb.

hand transfer with further evolution into vascularized joint transfer by 1976.[78] Free microvascular transfer of large volumes of tissue was accomplished in 1971 with Mclean and Buncke[79] transferring an omental flap to a skull defect. Shortly thereafter, Daniel and Taylor[80] accomplished the first microvascular extremity reconstruction by free transfer of a groin flap to the foot. Harii and colleagues[81] of Japan subsequently performed the first microvascular fasciocutaneous transfer in the upper extremity with a groin flap to the hand in 1973. The first free musculocutaneous transfers to the upper extremity were performed in 1976 by surgeons in China transferring pectoralis to the forearm (unknown to the world until subsequent years)[82] and Ikuta and colleagues[83] of Japan transferring gracilis to the forearm, both for treating Volkmann ischemic contractures by placing free-functioning muscle. The evolution of higher rungs of the reconstructive ladder of reconstruction in the upper extremity had progressed ahead of the development of the lower rungs with these microvascular transfers to the upper extremity occurring before the development of pedicled axially patterned fasciocutaneous,

musculocutaneous, and muscle flaps in the upper extremity.

Free flaps would now permeate the body using various tissues as donors and recipients. Taylor and colleagues[84] Tamai[85] introduced the fibular osseous and iliac osteocutaneous flaps in 1975 and 1976 respectively, and by 1979 these flaps were being used routinely in the upper extremity.[86] The upper extremity even evolved into a free flap donor site with the radial forearm flap performed by G.F. Yang of China in 1979.[87,88] The microsurgical progress in the People's Republic of China in the 1970s remained unknown to the rest of the world until an international delegation visited China in 1980, overcoming the political communication barrier. Hallock[89] introduced chimeric flaps (multiple different flaps harvested on the same source vessel) in 1991, and these flaps have provided effective coverage for mangled upper extremities with composite tissue requirements. Honda and colleagues[90] and Tsai and colleagues[91] first designed venous flow-through flaps for small defects of the hand in the 1980s. These venous flaps have been used in both free and pedicled fashions,[92–95] but they have remained less popular tools. The most recent iterations of free flaps include the free FDMA flap[96–98] introduced by Günter Germann in 1995 and the medial femoral condyle flap introduced by Doi and colleagues[99] in 2000. The latest evolutionary branch point, the composite tissue allograft, was first attempted in 1964, resulting in failure within 3 weeks caused by acute rejection.[100] The first successful hand transplantation occurred in 1998. Transplantation programs and pharmacologic treatments are still being optimized.[101]

Pedicled Muscle and Myocutaneous Flaps

The use of pedicled muscle flaps in the upper extremity is notable in that it represents a use of new anatomic knowledge from McCraw and colleagues[107] in an application of established principles to treat the traditional problem of plastic surgery: wounds of various causes. Thus, the accessibility of medical knowledge and literature was the greatest contributing factor enabling the evolution of these flaps, which can be traced most closely to the tissue transposition concepts of early plastic surgery. Stark[102] performed the first muscle transposition flaps by using the well-vascularized muscle on arms, thighs, and legs to treat osteomyelitis in 1946. However, Stark's[102] method did not become immediately popular. Years later, Ger[103–105] popularized the muscle flap in the late 1960s with his posterior leg compartment muscle flaps for covering tibial wounds. Drawing on his knowledge of muscle flap transpositions, Ger[106] introduced the brachioradialis transposition flap for reconstruction of a soft tissue defect from vascular surgical repair with exposed brachial artery in 1976. The next advance for muscle flaps came with McCraw and colleagues[107] elucidating the vascularity of these myocutaneous flaps in 1977. The gamut of pedicled muscle flaps for reconstruction of the upper extremity defects were developed during the 1980s and 1990s. Chase and colleagues[108] even described intrinsic hand muscle flaps using a myocutaneous adductor digiti minimi flap for both functional and soft tissue reconstruction of a thumb vascular malformation in 1980.

Third-generation Intrinsic Hand Flaps

Through the 1970s and 1980s, intrinsic hand flaps evolved their third-generation features with the pedicled island flaps, on which surgeons tested the limits of a skeletonized axial blood supply. These flaps were often designed to provide an innervated result on healing. The main evolutionary factor during this period is the arrival of a comprehensive catalog of published medical literature in

the newly revamped Index Medicus by the National Library of Medicine in 1960.[109] Access to previous techniques inspired the new innovations, as shown in the bibliographies of the published work of this era. The previous generation's dorsal transposition flaps were developed into sensate homodigital island flaps by Joshi.[110] The thumb dorsal transposition flap was similarly developed into a homodigital island flap by Pho.[111] Heterodigital island flap strategies combined the pedicled reinnervation concepts of Moberg and Littler with the spare parts (fillet flap) reconstructive methods of Peacock.[112–114] This period of time also saw further modification of the cross-finger concept producing the adipofascial cross-finger flap, which led to further homodigital use of the adipofascial turndown.[115,116]

1990 TO THE 2010S
Perforator/Free-style Flaps Developed from Anatomic Insights

The most recent major evolutionary branch of flap reconstructive technique, the perforator flaps, arose in the late 1980s. At that time, the knowledge accumulated by free flap surgeons in combination with anatomic studies allowed this breakthrough. The studies of Carl Manchot, Michel Salmon, and Ian Taylor had depicted cutaneous circulation emanating from larger source vessels within deeper layers of fascia and muscle. Carl Manchot had performed the first studies of this type in 1889 with his injection of vessels to investigate the anatomy of both cutaneous circulation and innervation, although his technique is not clear.[3,117–119] These studies were advanced in 1936 by French anatomist Michel Salmon who was able to show in great detail much smaller vessels than were shown by Manchot by his modified technique of intra-arterial injection of radio-opaque liquid and extensive use of radiography.[120] These studies were the foundation of the most recent investigations and descriptions of angiosomes by Ian Taylor. With these studies, Taylor provided the detailed maps for the concept that had challenged free flap surgeons for years: the arborized vascular supply of skin and fascia that emanates from various points of perforating vessels from a main pedicle, as described by Wei and colleagues[121] in 1986. These fundamental conceptual breakthroughs allowed the first perforator flap in 1989 with Koshima and Soeda[122] using the deep inferior epigastric artery perforator flaps to reconstruct extirpations of malignancy from the groin and tongue. In the upper extremity, the perforator flap concept has manifested with the lateral arm, posterior interosseous artery, ulnar artery, and radial artery perforator flaps.[123] In 2003, Fu-Chan Wei and Samir Mardini introduced a free-style technique of dissecting the vasculature of perforator flaps in retrograde fashion to be used in either pedicled or free flaps to allow an unparalleled tailoring of flap reconstruction to particular defects, especially in the upper extremity where minimizing the donor site defect is mandatory.[124–128]

Fourth-generation Intrinsic Hand Flaps and the Information Revolution

The most recent era of this history of upper extremity free flap reconstruction begins with the information revolution. Internet access has become ubiquitous in developed countries. Extensive literature searches that previously required days of being physically present at a major university library could now occur in minutes in the comfort of the clinician's own home with an Internet portal. This unprecedented access to the technical detail of previously published literature is the major evolutionary influence of this era. The technical innovations that arrived during this time show a unique creativity that can be seen with the fourth generation of intrinsic hand flaps (see **Fig. 2**). These flaps challenged the limits of previously established modalities and combined multiple flap reconstructive principles into individual techniques. Awf Quaba and Yu Maruyama used the unique pattern of vascularity in the hand to support the previous design of the FDMA-based flaps in a reversed vascular orientation similar to reversed-flow fasciocutaneous flaps on the limbs.[129–131] Furthermore, vascular islands and adipofascial flaps were viable when oriented on reversed flow on the fingers or on the palm.[132–136] Most recently, flaps have arisen such as the spiral flap, which resembles the Orticochea scalp flaps based on the unique axial blood supply of the hand.[137] The Gigone flap harnesses an island pedicle-based axial supply in a double V-Y advancement reminiscent of Atasoy's concept.[138] Boomerang flaps combine the concepts of reversed flow and perforator flaps.[139] Even smaller and more technically challenging island flaps have arisen with the digital artery perforator flaps.[140] These flaps combine principles in a way that is not seen elsewhere on the body.

The Future: Evidence-based Practice

The first major rate-limiting factor of evolution, the availability of information, has now become the major factor driving the continued evolution of upper extremity flap reconstruction. Surgical literature detailing each innovative technique is now widely available, and a wide arsenal of surgical techniques is available for reconstructing nearly every defect. With so many tools in the arsenal for upper extremity flap reconstruction, the next major challenge, with which surgeons have been grappling for the last 2 decades, is how most effectively to implement the surgical options for upper extremity flap reconstruction. The greatest factor influencing the evolution of upper extremity flap reconstruction in this regard is the evidence-based medicine movement, which gained momentum in the 1990s. Evidence-based recommendations now govern parameters of upper extremity reconstructive outcomes such as flap loss, infection, bone healing, donor site morbidity, length of hospital stay, economics, and aesthetics. Flap choice, reconstructive timing, wound factors, surgeon factors, and patient factors have all been queried as input variables. However, various flap reconstructions on the hand are difficult to study because the significant injuries of the hand involve a complex combination of skeletal, tendon, and nerve injuries. Therefore, it is difficult to make functional assessments on just the reconstructive modality alone. Furthermore, assessing tissue healing as an outcome variable of these surgeries is also subject to numerous uncontrolled variables of injury. There are also unsolved challenges that present themselves for upper extremity flap reconstruction. Severe cicatricial burn scarring causing impaired tendon gliding and disabling joint contracture has not found suitable reconstruction by either conventional skin grafting or more extensive excisions with flap reconstruction. The end-stage mangled hand similarly finds limited functional benefit from upper extremity flap reconstruction. Both of these disorders seem destined to be managed by composite tissue allotransplantation in the future. Vascularized groin lymph node flap transfers with progressively smaller anastomotic targets (supermicrosurgery) are on the frontier of hand surgery and plastic surgery, and outcomes analyses are still indeterminate as to the success of this technique.[141,142] In future, these new techniques of upper extremity flap reconstruction will evolve more quickly because the factors that drive this process (access to surgical technique and interchange of ideas) have become well integrated into current surgical practice. The clinical outcome of the reconstructions will increasingly be the major factor that drives the direction of this evolution.

REFERENCES

1. Greco M, Ciriaco AG, Vonella M, et al. The primacy of the Vianeo family in the invention of nasal

reconstruction technique. Ann Plast Surg 2010; 64(6):702–5.

2. Choulant L, Frank M. History and bibliography of anatomic illustration. New York: Hafner Publishing; 1962.

3. Santoni-Rugiu P, Sykes PJ. A history of plastic surgery. Berlin, London: Springer; 2007.

4. Cox C, Yao J. Electrocautery use in hand surgery: history, physics, and appropriate usage. J Hand Surg 2010;35(3):489–90.

5. Trunkey DD. The emerging crisis in trauma care: a history and definition of the problem. Clin Neurosurg 2007;54:200–5.

6. Lee MR. The history of Ephedra (ma-huang). J R Coll Physicians Edinb 2011;41(1):78–84.

7. Kragh JF Jr, Swan KG, Smith DC, et al. Historical review of emergency tourniquet use to stop bleeding. Am J Surg 2012;203(2):242–52.

8. Cooper BB, Bransby B. Cooper's lectures on amputation. Boston Med Surg J 1849;41(16):309–14.

9. Kirkup J. A history of limb amputation. London: Springer; 2007.

10. Loimer H, Guarnieri M. Accidents and acts of God: a history of the terms. Am J Public Health 1996; 86(1):101–7.

11. Musson AA, Robinson E. Science and technology in the industrial revolution, vol. 3. London: Gordon and Breach; 1969.

12. Helling TS, Daon E. In Flanders fields: the Great War, Antoine Depage, and the resurgence of debridement. Ann Surg 1998;228(2):173–81.

13. Davis WC. Fighting for time. Volume 4, the image of war, 1861–1865. Garden City (NY): Doubleday; 1983.

14. United States Surgeon General's Office, Otis GA, Barnes JK. The medical and surgical history of the war of the rebellion: surgical history. Washington, DC: Government Printing Office; 2011.

15. Bentley R. Different roads to discovery; Prontosil (hence sulfa drugs) and penicillin (hence beta-lactams). J Ind Microbiol Biotechnol 2009;36(6): 775–86.

16. Giangrande PL. The history of blood transfusion. Br J Haematol 2000;110(4):758–67.

17. Noe A. Extremity injury in war: a brief history. J Am Acad Orthop Surg 2006;14(Spec No 10):S1–6.

18. Jeffrey H. Blood transfusion in war. J R Army Med Corps 1974;120(1):24–30.

19. Shrady G. The finger as a medium for transplanting skin flaps. Med Rec 1891;39:117.

20. Halsted W. Plastic operation for extensive burn of neck. Bull Johns Hopkins Hosp 1896;25.

21. Hamilton FH. Elkoplasty; or, anaplasty applied to the treatment of old ulcers: also, a new mode of treatment for delayed or non-union of a fractured humerus. New York: Holman Gray; 1854.

22. Stark RB, Kaplan JM. Cross-leg flaps in patients over 50 years of age. Br J Plast Surg 1972;25:20–1.

23. Baux GS, Fischer E, McCarthy JG. Frank Hastings Hamilton: a pioneer American plastic surgeon. Plast Reconstr Surg 2004;114(5):1240–7.

24. Wood J. Case of extreme deformity of the neck and forearm, from the cicatrices of a burn, cured by extension, excision, and transplantation of skin, adjacent and remote. Med Chir Trans 1863;46:149.

25. Roberts JB. Salvage of the hand by timely reparative surgery. Ann Surg 1919;70(5):627.

26. Maxwell GP. Iginio Tansini and the origin of the latissimus dorsi musculocutaneous flap. Plast Reconstr Surg 1980;65(5):686–92.

27. Teimourian B, Adham MN. Louis Ombredanne and the origin of muscle flap use for immediate breast mound reconstruction. Plast Reconstr Surg 1983; 72(6):905–10.

28. Gurunluoglu R, Shafighi M, Huemer GM, et al. Carl Nicoladoni (1847–1902): professor of surgery. Ann Surg 2004;239(2):281.

29. The classic: plastic surgery of the thumb and organic substitution of the fingertip (anticheiroplastic surgery and finger plastic surgery). By Carl Nicoladoni, 1900. Clin Orthop Relat Res 1985;195:3–6.

30. Joyce BM. A new operation for the substitution of a thumb. Br J Surg 1917;5(19):499–504.

31. Joyce JL. The results of a new operation for the substitution of a thumb. Br J Surg 1929;16(63): 362–9.

32. Albee FH. Synthetic transplantation of tissues to form new finger: with restored function of hand. Ann Surg 1919;69(4):379.

33. Chambers JA, Davis MR, Rasmussen TE. A band of surgeons, a long healing line: development of craniofacial surgery in response to armed conflict. J Craniofac Surg 2010;21(4):991–7.

34. Davis JS. Plastic surgery in World War I and in World War II. Plast Reconstr Surg 1946;1(3):255–64.

35. Chambers JA, Ray PD. Achieving growth and excellence in medicine: the case history of armed conflict and modern reconstructive surgery. Ann Plast Surg 2009;63(5):473–8.

36. Bunnell S, Coates JB. Hand surgery in World War II. Office of the Surgeon-General, Department of the Army. 1955.

37. Howard LD Jr. Hand surgery. AMA Arch Surg 1960; 80(3):374–8.

38. Myers G. A study of the causes of industrial accidents. Q Publ Am Stat Assoc 1915;14(111): 672–94.

39. Gatewood J. A plastic repair of finger defects without hospitalization. JAMA 1926;87:1479.

40. Shaw DT, Payne R Jr. One stage tubed abdominal flaps; single pedicle tubes. Surg Gynecol Obstet 1946;83:205.

41. DeJongh E. A simple plastic procedure of the fingers for conserving bony tissue and forming a soft tissue pad. Am J Surg 1942;57(2):346–7.

42. Kutler W. A new method for finger tip amputation. J Am Med Assoc 1947;133(1):29–30.

43. Geissendörfer H. Beitrag zur Fingerkuppenplastik. Zentralbl Chir 1943;70:1107–8.

44. Heinrich HW, Petersen D, Roos N. Industrial accident prevention. New York: McGraw-Hill; 1950.

45. Gudin M, Pangman WJ. The repair of surface defects of fingers by trans-digital flaps. Plast Reconstr Surg 1950;5(4):368.

46. Cronin TD. The cross finger flap: a new method of repair. Am Surg 1951;17(5):419.

47. Lewin ML. Digital flaps. Plast Reconstr Surg 1951; 7(1):46–9.

48. Flatt AE. Minor hand injuries. J Bone Joint Surg Br 1955;37(1):117.

49. Hilgenfeldt O. Operativer daumenersatz. Stuttgart (Germany): Enke; 1950.

50. Holevich J. A new method of restoring sensibility to the thumb. J Bone Joint Surg Br 1963;45:496.

51. Foucher G, Braun J-B. A new island flap transfer from the dorsum of the index to the thumb. Plast Reconstr Surg 1979;63(3):344–9.

52. Vilain R. Technique élémentaire de réparation des pertes de substance cutanée des doigts. Sem Hop Paris 1952;28:1223–7.

53. Iselin F. The flag flap. Plast Reconstr Surg 1973; 52(4):374–7.

54. Lister G. Local flaps to the hand. Hand Clin 1985; 1(4):621.

55. O'Brien B. Neurovascular island pedicle flaps for terminal amputations and digital scars. Br J Plast Surg 1968;21(2):258–61.

56. Snow JW. The use of a volar flap for repair of fingertip amputations: a preliminary report. Plast Reconstr Surg 1967;40(2):163–8.

57. Moberg E. Aspects of sensation in reconstructive surgery of the upper extremity. J Bone Joint Surg Am 1964;46(4):817–25.

58. Lueders HW, Shapiro RL. Rotation finger flaps in reconstruction of burned hands. Plast Reconstr Surg 1971;47(2):176–8.

59. Joshi BB. Dorsolateral flap from same finger to relieve flexion contracture. Plast Reconstr Surg 1972;49(2):186–9.

60. Smith P. A sliding flap to cover dorsal skin defects over the proximal interphalangeal joint. Hand 1982; 14(3):271–8.

61. Ogunro O. Dorsal transposition flap for reconstruction of lateral or medial oblique amputations of the thumb with exposure of bone. J Hand Surg 1983; 8(6):894–8.

62. Inoue G. Fingertip reconstruction with a dorsal transposition flap. Br J Plast Surg 1991;44(7): 530–2.

63. Flint MH, Harrison SH. A local neurovascular flap to repair loss of the digital pulp. Br J Plast Surg 1965; 18:156–63.

64. Levame J, Otero C, Berdugo G. Vascularisation artérielle des téguments de la face dorsale de la main et des doigts. Ann Chir Plast 1967;12: 316–24.

65. Flint MH. Some observations on the vascular supply of the nail bed and terminal segments of the finger. Br J Plast Surg 1955;8(0):186–95.

66. Hueston J. Local flap repair of fingertip injuries. Plast Reconstr Surg 1966;37(4):349–50.

67. Atasoy E, Ioakimidis E, Kasdan ML, et al. Reconstruction of the amputated finger tip with a triangular volar flap a new surgical procedure. J Bone Joint Surg Am 1970;52(5):921–6.

68. McCash CR. Cross-arm bridge flaps in the repair of flexion contractures of the fingers. Br J Plast Surg 1957;9:25–33.

69. Von Deilen AW, Coxau JB. Immediate replacement of tissue losses from hand or wrist by means of bipedicled cross arm flaps. Am J Surg 1957;94(5): 790–3.

70. McGregor IA, Jackson IT. The extended role of the delto-pectoral flap. Br J Plast Surg 1970; 23(0):173–85.

71. Kriss TC, Kriss VM. History of the operating microscope: from magnifying glass to microneurosurgery. Neurosurgery 1998;42(4):899–907.

72. Malt RA, McKhann CF. Replantation of severed arms. JAMA 1964;189(10):716–22.

73. Kleinert HE, Kasdan ML, Romero JL. Small bloodvessel anastomosis for salvage of severely injured upper extremity. J Bone Joint Surg Am 1963;45(4): 788–96.

74. Kleinert HE, Kasdan ML. Anastamosis of digital vessels. J Ky Med Assoc 1965;63:106–8.

75. Yang D, Gu Y, Wu M. Thumb reconstruction by free second toe transplantation. Report of 40 cases. Zhonghua Wai Ke Za Zhi 1977;15(1):13–8.

76. Dongyue Y, Yudong G. Thumb reconstruction utilizing second toe transplantation by microvascular anastomosis: report of 78 cases. Chin Med J 1979;92(5):295.

77. Cobbett J. Free digital transfer. J Bone Joint Surg Br 1969;51:677–9.

78. Foucher G, Merle M, Maneaud M, et al. Microsurgical free partial toe transfer in hand reconstruction: a report of 12 cases. Plast Reconstr Surg 1980;65(5):616–26.

79. Mclean DH, Buncke HJ Jr. Autotransplant of omentum to a large scalp defect, with microsurgical revascularization. Plast Reconstr Surg 1972;49(3): 268–74.

80. Daniel RK, Taylor GI. Distant transfer of an island flap by microvascular anastomoses. Plast Reconstr Surg 1973;52(2):111–7.

81. Harii K, Ohmori K, Ohmori S. Successful clinical transfer of ten free flaps by microvascular anastomoses. Plast Reconstr Surg 1974;53(3):259–70.

82. Free muscle transplantation by microsurgical neurovascular anastomoses. Report of a case. Chin Med J 1976;2(1):47–50.

83. Ikuta Y, Kubo T, Tsuge K. Free muscle transplantation by microsurgical technique to treat severe Volkmann's contracture. Plast Reconstr Surg 1976;58(4):407–11.

84. Taylor GI, Miller GD, Ham FJ. The free vascularized bone graft: a clinical extension of microvascular techniques. Plast Reconstr Surg 1975;55(5): 533–44.

85. Tamai S. Iliac osteocutaneous neurosensory flap. Microsurgical composite tissue transplantation. St Louis (MO): Mosby; 1979. p. 391–7.

86. Weiland AJ, Kleinert HE, Kutz JE, et al. Free vascularized bone grafts in surgery of the upper extremity. J Hand Surg 1979;4(2):129–44.

87. Yang GF, Chen PJ, Gao YZ, et al. Forearm free skin flap transplantation: a report of 56 cases. Br J Plast Surg 1997;50(3):162–5.

88. Boo-Chai K. Some notes on Dr Yang Guo-Fan, MD, and the forearm free flap. Plast Reconstr Surg 1997;99(3):919–21.

89. Hallock GG. Simultaneous transposition of anterior thigh muscle and fascia flaps: an introduction to the chimera flap principle. Ann Plast Surg 1991; 27(2):126–31.

90. Honda T, Yamauchi S, Shimamura K, et al. The possible applications of a composite skin and subcutaneous vein graft in the replantation of amputated digits. Br J Plast Surg 1984;37(4): 607–12.

91. Tsai T-M, Matiko JD, Breidenbach W, et al. Venous flaps in digital revascularization and replantation. J Reconstr Microsurg 1987;3(02):113–9.

92. Chavoin J, Rouge D, Vachaud M, et al. Island flaps with an exclusively venous pedicle. A report of eleven cases and a preliminary haemodynamic study. Br J Plast Surg 1987;40(2):149–54.

93. Foucher G, Norris R. The venous dorsal digital island flap or the "neutral" flap. Br J Plast Surg 1988;41(4):337–43.

94. Kayikçioglu A, Akyürek M, Safak T, et al. Arterialized venous dorsal digital island flap for fingertip reconstruction. Plast Reconstr Surg 1998;102(7): 2368–72.

95. Inada Y, Fukui A, Tamai S, et al. The sliding venous flap for covering skin defects with poor blood supply on the lateral aspects of fingers. Br J Plast Surg 1991;44(5):368–71.

96. Germann G, Hornung R, Raff T. Two new applications for the first dorsal metacarpal artery pedicle in the treatment of severe hand injuries. J Hand Surg Br 1995;20(4):525–8.

97. Inoue T, Ueda K, Kurihara T, et al. A new cutaneous flap: snuff-box flap. Br J Plast Surg 1993;46(3): 252–4.

98. Takamatsu A, Inoue T, Kurihara T, et al. Free snuff-box flap for reconstruction of the wrap-around flap donor site. Br J Plast Surg 1995;48(5):312–7.

99. Doi K, Oda T, Soo-Heong T, et al. Free vascularized bone graft for nonunion of the scaphoid. J Hand Surg 2000;25(3):507–19.

100. Gilbert R. Transplant is successful with a cadaver forearm. Med Trib Med News 1964;5:20.

101. Dubernard JM, Owen E, Herzberg G, et al. Human hand allograft: report on first 6 months. Lancet 1999;353(9161):1315–20.

102. Stark W. The use of pedicled muscle flaps in the surgical treatment of chronic osteomyelitis resulting from compound fractures. J Bone Joint Surg Am 1946;28(2):343–50.

103. Ger R. The operative treatment of the advanced stasis ulcer: a preliminary communication. Am J Surg 1966;111(5):659–63.

104. Ger R. The management of pretibial skin loss. Surgery 1968;63(5):757–63.

105. Ger R, Efron G. New operative approach in the treatment of chronic osteomyelitis of the tibial diaphysis: a preliminary report. Clin Orthop Relat Res 1970;70:165–9.

106. Ger R. The coverage of vascular repairs by muscle transposition. J Trauma 1976;16(12):974–8.

107. McCraw JB, Dibbell DG, Carraway JH. Clinical definition of independent myocutaneous vascular territories. Plast Reconstr Surg 1977;60(3):341–52.

108. Chase RA, Hentz VR, Apfelberg D. A dynamic myocutaneous flap for hand reconstruction. J Hand Surg 1980;5(6):594–9.

109. Lipscomb CE. Medical subject headings (MeSH). Bull Med Libr Assoc 2000;88(3):265.

110. Joshi BB. A local dorsolateral island flap for restoration of sensation after avulsion injury of fingertip pulp. Plast Reconstr Surg 1974;54(2):175–82.

111. Pho R. Restoration of sensation using a local neurovascular island flap as a primary procedure in extensive pulp loss of the fingertip. Injury 1976; 8(1):20–4.

112. Peacock EE Jr. Reconstruction of the hand by the local transfer of composite tissue island flaps. Plast Reconstr Surg 1960;25(4):298–311.

113. Rose EH. Local arterialized island flap coverage of difficult hand defects preserving donor digit sensibility. Plast Reconstr Surg 1983;72(6):848–57.

114. Tubiana R, Duparc J. Restoration of sensibility in the hand by neurovascular skin island transfer. J Bone Joint Surg Br 1961;43(3):474–80.

115. Ivan Pakiam A. The reversed dermis flap. Br J Plast Surg 1978;31(2):131–5.

116. Thatte RL, Gopalakrishna A, Prasad S. The use of de-epithelialised "turn over" flaps in the hand. Br J Plast Surg 1982;35(3):293–9.

117. Verdan C. The history of hand surgery in Europe. J Hand Surg Br 2000;25(3):238–41.

118. Manchot C. Die Hautarterien des menschlichen Körpers. London: Vogel; 1889.

119. Manchot C, Ristic J. The cutaneous arteries of the human body. New York: Springer-Verlag; 1983.

120. Cormack GC, Lamberty BG. The arterial anatomy of skin flaps. Edinburgh (United Kingdom): Churchill Livingstone; 1994.

121. Wei FC, Chen HC, Chuang CC, et al. Fibular osteoseptocutaneous flap: anatomic study and clinical application. Plast Reconstr Surg 1986;78(2):191–9.

122. Koshima I, Soeda S. Inferior epigastric artery skin flaps without rectus abdominis muscle. Br J Plast Surg 1989;42(6):645–8.

123. Blondeel P, Morris S, Neligan P, et al. Perforator flaps: anatomy, techniques and clinical applications. 2005.

124. Mardini S, Tsai FC, Wei FC. The thigh as a model for free style free flaps. Clin Plast Surg 2003; 30(3):473–80.

125. Wei FC, Mardini S. Free-style free flaps. Plast Reconstr Surg 2004;114(4):910–6.

126. Wallace CG, Kao HK, Jeng SF, et al. Free-style flaps: a further step forward for perforator flap surgery. Plast Reconstr Surg 2009;124(6S):e419–26.

127. Lecours C, Saint-Cyr M, Wong C, et al. Freestyle pedicle perforator flaps: clinical results and vascular anatomy. Plast Reconstr Surg 2010; 126(5):1589–603.

128. D'Arpa S, Cordova A, Pignatti M, et al. Freestyle pedicled perforator flaps: safety, prevention of complications, and management based on 85 consecutive cases. Plast Reconstr Surg 2011; 128(4):892–906.

129. Quaba A, Davison P. The distally-based dorsal hand flap. Br J Plast Surg 1990;43(1):28–39.

130. Maruyama Y. The reverse dorsal metacarpal flap. Br J Plast Surg 1990;43(1):24–7.

131. Brunelli F, Pegin Z, Cabral J. Dorsal arterial supply to the thumb. Surg Radiol Anat 1991;13(3):240–2.

132. Omokawa S, Yajima H, Inada Y, et al. A reverse ulnar hypothenar flap for finger reconstruction. Plast Reconstr Surg 2000;106(4):828–33.

133. Zancolli E. Colgajo cutaneo en isla del hueco de la palma. Prensa Med Argent 1990;77:14–20.

134. Oberlin C, Sarcy JJ, Alnot JY. Apport artériel cutané de la main. Application à la réalisation des lambeaux en îlot. Annales de Chirurgie de la Main, Vol. 7. No. 2. Ile de: Elsevier Masson; 1988.

135. Lai CS, Lin SD, Yang CC. The reverse digital artery flap for fingertip reconstruction. Ann Plast Surg 1989;22(6):495–500.

136. Chang KP, Wang WH, Lai CS, et al. Refinement of reverse digital arterial flap for finger defects: surgical technique. J Hand Surg 2005;30(3):558–61.

137. Lim GJ, Yam AK, Lee JY, et al. The spiral flap for fingertip resurfacing: short-term and long-term results. J Hand Surg 2008;33(3):340–7.

138. Bakhach J, Guimberteau J, Panconi B. The Gigogne flap: an original technique for an optimal pulp reconstruction. J Hand Surg Eur Vol 2009; 34(2):227–34.

139. Chen SL, Chou TD, Chen SG, et al. The boomerang flap in managing injuries of the dorsum of the distal phalanx. Plast Reconstr Surg 2000;106(4):834–9.

140. Koshima I, Urushibara K, Fukuda N, et al. Digital artery perforator flaps for fingertip reconstructions. Plast Reconstr Surg 2006;118(7):1579–84.

141. Lin CH, Ali R, Chen SC, et al. Vascularized groin lymph node transfer using the wrist as a recipient site for management of postmastectomy upper extremity lymphedema. Plast Reconstr Surg 2009; 123(4):1265–75.

142. Cheng MH, Chen SC, Henry SL, et al. Vascularized groin lymph node flap transfer for postmastectomy upper limb lymphedema: flap anatomy, recipient sites, and outcomes. Plast Reconstr Surg 2013; 131(6):1286–98.

Anatomy and Physiology of Perforator Flaps of the Upper Limb

Sarah E. Appleton, MD, MSc[a],
Steven F. Morris, MD, MSc, FRCSC[b],*

KEYWORDS

- Upper extremity • Radial artery perforator flap • Ulnar artery perforator flap
- Posterior interosseous artery flap • Lateral arm flap • First dorsal metacarpal artery perforator flap
- Perforator-based propeller flap

KEY POINTS

- A functional result is of foremost importance in upper limb reconstruction.
- Perforator flaps are an excellent reconstructive option for a functional upper limb reconstruction.
- Principles of flap surgery include the transfer of similar tissue with the least donor site morbidity in a single stage procedure.
- A thorough understanding of cutaneous perforator anatomy significantly increases the reconstructive options for the upper limb.
- Perforator-based propeller flaps are a versatile option for upper limb reconstruction.

INTRODUCTION

What is a Perforator Flap?

There are many different types and classifications of perforator flaps. A perforator flap is a flap consisting of skin and/or subcutaneous fat based on one or more vascular tributaries of a single source artery. Small vessels supplying blood to the flap are termed *perforators*. Perforators arise from a source vessel and pass either through (indirect) or between (direct) deeper tissues (ie, muscle) to supply the skin. A septocutaneous perforator transverses only through septum to supply the overlying skin after piercing the outer layers of the deep fascia.[1] A muscle or musculocutaneous perforator courses through muscle and pierces the outer layer of deep fascia to supply the overlying skin.[1] Some perforator flaps are flaps that are familiar and commonly used. Others have evolved based on the perforator flap concept, are not commonly used, and have not reached all surgeons. In general, perforator flaps may be used in 3 major ways: pedicled flaps, transposition flaps, and free tissue flaps.[2] A propeller flap is a uniquely designed transposition-type perforator flap based on a single dissected perforator.[3] The flap is designed in a propeller shape with 2 blades of unequal length with the perforator located at a central pivot point. The blades are rotated up to 180° to allow the long propeller arm to fill the defect.[4] The propeller flap has been used reliably in trauma reconstruction of the lower limb in particular (**Fig. 1**).[5]

Funding Sources: Nil.
Conflicts of Interest: Nil.
[a] Plastic and Reconstructive Surgery, Dalhousie University, 4443-1796 Summer Street, Halifax, Nova Scotia B3H 3A7, Canada; [b] Departments of Surgery, Anatomy and Neurobiology, Dalhousie University, 4443-1796 Summer Street, Halifax, Nova Scotia B3H 3A7, Canada
* Corresponding author.
E-mail address: sfmorris@dal.ca

Hand Clin 30 (2014) 123–135
http://dx.doi.org/10.1016/j.hcl.2013.12.003
0749-0712/14/$ – see front matter © 2014 Elsevier Inc. All rights reserved.

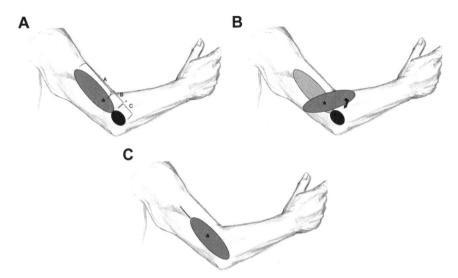

Fig. 1. The perforator propeller flap concept. The perforator (*red star*) is the hub of the propeller and the pivot point of the flap composed of 2 asymmetric limbs. (*A*) The distance from the perforator to the distal edge of the wound (B + C) equals slightly less than the length of the proximal, longer limb (A) of the flap. (*B, C*) When rotated 180°, the longer limb (A) rotates to fill the defect.

Upper Extremity Reconstruction

There are many indications for the use of perforator flaps in the upper extremity.[6] In general, the simplest strategy to obtain problem-free wound healing and early mobilization is optimal for upper extremity reconstruction. Ideal wounds suitable for flap reconstruction in the upper extremity often have exposed joint, bone, tendon or nerve, or extensive combined defects. The defects may be found in an area in which a skin graft may be unstable and lead to wound breakdown. Perforator flaps are ideal in areas where further surgery is likely or to cover massive wounds with significant soft tissue loss. A skin flap is far superior to a muscle flap when reoperation is likely because skin revascularizes very quickly, whereas muscle revascularizes slowly and incompletely. Also, skin reconstruction has a superior aesthetic appearance compared with skin-grafted muscle.

The improved understanding of the vascular anatomy of the skin of the upper limb has increased the available flap options for upper extremity reconstruction. In the past, random flaps and 2-staged pedicle flaps were used to reconstruct the upper limb with suboptimal functional outcomes. Pedicled flaps, such as the groin flap, delay definitive reconstruction, cause additional surgical stages, promote stiffness, and usually lead to inferior results. Now there are numerous reconstructive options using local pedicled perforator flaps, regional perforator flaps, and free tissue transfers. Today, musculocutaneous flaps have been largely replaced by free skin flaps or regional perforator flaps for the optimal functional upper limb reconstruction.

ANATOMY

A thorough understanding of the vascular anatomy of the upper limb is essential to the success of free tissue transfers in this region. The main source vessel to the upper limb is the brachial artery. The axillary artery supplies branches only to the shoulder region. Blood supply to forearm skin is provided by the cutaneous branches of the brachial artery as well as the musculocutaneous and septocutaneous perforators of the radial and ulnar arteries.[7] Direct fasciocutaneous perforators from the radial, ulnar, anterior, and posterior interosseous arteries supply most of the forearm.[7] The ulnar artery supplies the palmar hand via the superficial palmar arch. The dorsal metacarpal arteries from the radial artery supply the dorsum of the hand. The distal third of the forearm has more numerous small-caliber perforators, whereas the proximal forearm has fewer larger-caliber perforator vessels that branch over a larger surface area. The distal forearm tends to lend itself to smaller flaps, and the proximal forearm can usually support a larger flap based on a single perforator vessel. As a general rule, the dominant cutaneous vessels of the upper extremity perforate the deep fascia at fixed sites within the intermuscular septa or the major intramuscular septa.[8]

Perforating cutaneous vessels can be reliably traced back to one source vessel (**Fig. 2, Table 1**).

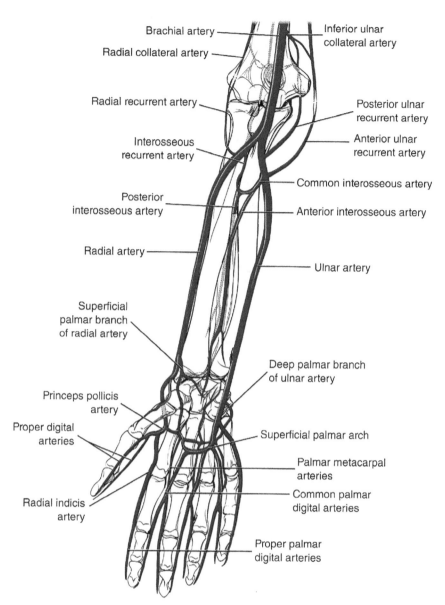

Fig. 2. Arterial anatomy of the upper limb. (*From* Morris SF, Gupta A, Saint-Cyr M. Chapter 55: flap options and technical considerations in the upper extremity. In: Blondeel PN, Morris SF, Hallock GG, et al, editors. Perforator flaps: anatomy, technique and clinical applications. 2nd edition. St Louis (MO): Quality Medical Publishing; copyright 2013. p. 960; with permission.)

This factor becomes important when searching for recipient vessels adjacent to a soft tissue defect. The body can be divided into anatomic territories or angiosomes composed of composite blocks of tissue supplied by a source artery and linked together by anastomotic vessels spanning skin and bone (**Fig. 3**).[9,10] Cutaneous skin angiosomes of the body are linked together like a patchwork quilt. Research has demonstrated that the clinical territory of a cutaneous perforator extends outward in all directions to encompass the anatomic territory of adjacent angiosomes.[11,12] We can use the angiosome theory and this knowledge to design larger flaps safely.[1,12]

Variations in human anatomy have been noted since the earliest anatomic studies. The design of local perforator flaps depends on the identification of a suitable perforator adjacent to the defect. Preoperative computed tomography angiograms may be useful for surgical planning if available because variation in human vascular anatomy is relatively common.[13,14] The use of a Doppler

Table 1
Cutaneous vascular territories of the upper extremity by arterial vessel source

Source Artery	Branches
Axillary artery	Acromial branches of suprascapular ± thoracoacromial arteries (TAA) Deltoid branch of thoracoacromial artery Anterior circumflex humeral artery Posterior circumflex humeral artery (PCHA)
Brachial artery (BA)	Direct musculocutaneous and septocutaneous branches Profunda brachial artery (PBA) • Radial collateral artery ○ Posterior radial collateral artery (PRCA) • Middle collateral artery Superior ulnar collateral artery (SUCA) Inferior ulnar collateral (supratrochlear) artery (IUCA)
Radial artery (RA)	Direct musculocutaneous and septocutaneous branches Radial recurrent artery (RRA) Superior palmar branch Deep palmar arch (DPA) • Princeps pollicis artery • Radialis indicis artery • Palmar metacarpal artery • Proper digital artery • Proper palmar digital artery Dorsal carpal arch (DCA) • Dorsal metacarpal arteries
Ulnar artery (UA)	Direct musculocutaneous and septocutaneous branches Anterior ulnar recurrent artery Posterior ulnar recurrent artery Common interosseous artery • Anterior interosseous artery (AIOA) • Posterior interosseous artery (PIOA) ○ Interosseous recurrent artery Superficial palmar arch (SPA) • Common palmar digital arteries • Proper palmar digital arteries Deep palmar arch (DPA) Dorsal metacarpal artery (DMA)

probe preoperatively to outline the perforators has also been shown to be useful.[1,14,15] Intraoperative direct visualization of perforators is also an excellent method that is frequently used to identify perforators.[1,16]

FLAP PHYSIOLOGY AND GENERAL PRINCIPLES

General principles of upper limb soft tissue reconstructive surgery are consistent with those applied elsewhere in the body. The need to accomplish a reconstruction that will promote optimal function is foremost in the reconstruction of a functional upper limb. The most reliable, efficient procedure should be used whenever possible; however, overtreatment should be avoided. Upper extremity trauma reconstruction should be planned with an emphasis on restoring form and function.[17] Often, the simplest method for obtaining wound closure may not lead to the best functional outcome. For example, a free tissue transfer with extensor tendon grafts in a one-stage reconstruction for an avulsion injury to the dorsum of the hand would offer a complete functional reconstruction, whereas a simple skin graft for wound closure would not.[18]

The best donor tissue available that can be harvested with the least donor-site morbidity and the highest chance of success should be used. The ideal tissue for any reconstruction should match the characteristics of the missing tissue in the area of the defect. The tissue type varies significantly by region in the upper extremity. In the fingers, tissue coverage must be thin and pliable, whereas palmar skin is glabrous, durable, and thick. Upper arm and forearm skin quality is variable. Whenever possible, reconstruction using adjacent tissues is usually preferable. Obesity influences flap choices because a thick flap will adversely affect extremity mobility.

Early or immediate reconstruction of upper extremity wounds after soft tissue trauma to the upper limb is usually indicated and advocated. Early reconstruction has been shown to improve the overall functional outcome of the reconstruction.[19,20] Upper limb structures are prone to desiccation, and early wound closure preserves the remaining tissues and prevents desiccation and infection. Immediate or early definitive soft tissue reconstruction has been shown to be superior when compared with delayed or multiple debridements followed by surgical reconstruction of the wound.[19–21] Reconstructive options that allow or promote early mobilization are essential in terms of rehabilitation. One-stage procedures are almost always preferred over multi-stage procedures

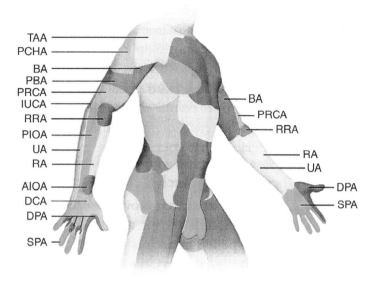

Fig. 3. Angiosomes of the upper limb. Vascular territories of the upper limb are shown in different colors. Each color corresponds to a different source artery. AIOA, anterior interosseous artery; BA, brachial artery; DCA, dorsal carpal arch; DPA, deep palmar arch; IUCA, inferior ulnar collateral artery; PBA, profunda brachial artery; PCHA, posterior circumflex humeral artery; PIOA, posterior interosseous artery; PRCA, posterior radial collateral artery; RA, radial artery; RRA, radial recurrent artery; SPA, superficial palmar arch; TAA, thoracoacromial arteries; UA, ulnar artery. Vascular territories are listed in **Table 1**. (*From* Yang D, Al Dhamin AS, Morris SF. Chapter 18: ulnar artery perforator flap. In: Blondeel PN, Morris SF, Hallock GG, et al, editors. Perforator flaps: anatomy, technique and clinical applications. 2nd edition. St Louis (MO): Quality Medical Publishing; copyright 2013. p.370; with permission.)

because results are superior and hospitalization and cost of care are reduced.

One of the main advantages of using perforator flaps is the ability to harvest skin flaps based on large source vessels. Patients undergoing reconstruction of extensive wounds in the upper extremity often do better with skin flaps when compared with muscle flaps. Skin or fasciocutaneous flaps also offer a better color and contour match for an improved aesthetic result. The rate of neovascularization of the transferred skin flap is faster than with muscle flaps.[22–24] Therefore, if a secondary procedure is needed in a skin or fasciocutaneous flap, it is less problematic. Incisions made through a muscle flap, even years later, may result in partial flap necrosis or wound breakdown.[24–26]

PERFORATOR FLAPS OF THE UPPER EXTREMITY

The goals of reconstruction of the upper extremity following soft tissue loss include the following: (1) salvaging the extremity, (2) early functional restoration, (3) individualized reconstruction, (4) an aesthetic outcome, and (5) cost-effective treatment.[18] There are a wide variety of perforator flap options that offer several choices for the surgeon performing reconstruction of the upper limb (**Table 2**). This article reviews in more detail the most essential perforator flaps in the reconstructive surgeon's toolbox for upper extremity trauma reconstruction. The flaps discussed include the

Table 2
Upper extremity perforator flaps by region

Region	Flap Options
Shoulder and upper arm	Posterior circumflex humeral artery flap (deltoid flap)
	Superior ulnar collateral artery flap (medial arm flap)
	Posterior radial collateral artery flap (lateral arm flap)
	Posterior upper arm flap (brachial artery)
Elbow	Inferior cubital artery flap
	Posterior interosseous recurrent artery flap
	Ulnar recurrent artery flap
	Reverse posterior radial collateral artery flap (lateral arm flap)
Forearm	**Radial artery perforator flap**
	Ulnar artery perforator flap
	Dorsal ulnar artery flap
	Flexor carpi ulnaris flap
	Brachioradialis flap
Hand	**First dorsal metacarpal artery**
	Dorsal ulnar thumb flap
	Second dorsal metacarpal artery flap
	Reverse dorsal metacarpal artery flap

Flaps discussed in greater detail identified in bold.

radial artery perforator, ulnar artery perforator, posterior interosseous perforator, lateral arm perforator, and the first dorsal metacarpal artery (FDMA) perforator flap. Any of these flaps can be customized in many ways depending on the particular application. Also, virtually any adequately sized perforator in the upper limb could be used for a local perforator free-style transfer.

Radial Artery Perforator Flap

The radial forearm perforator flap is a large, thin, versatile, well-vascularized flap commonly used to cover moderate sized (8–18 cm) hand and wrist defects.[27] It is most commonly used as a skin flap, but tendon (flexor carpi radialis), fascia (forearm fascia), bone (radius), and nerve (lateral antebrachial cutaneous nerve of the forearm) may be incorporated in the flap design as needed. The radial artery perforator flap may also be raised as a free flap or elevated based on the proximal radial artery perforators and rotated to cover proximal forearm or elbow defects (**Fig. 4**).

Vascular anatomy

The radial artery courses between the brachioradialis and flexor carpi radialis muscles to the radial styloid process and supplies the radial aspect of the forearm through a series of 15 to 25 perforators.[28,29] In the proximal forearm, the radial artery

courses deep between the brachioradialis and pronator teres muscles. In the distal forearm, the radial artery can be found more superficially between the brachioradialis and the flexor carpi radialis. At the level of the wrist, the radial artery passes deep to the abductor pollicis longus and extensor pollicis brevis tendons and continues into the anatomic snuffbox where it forms the deep palmar arch. Anatomic studies have reliably shown at least one large perforator in the proximal, middle, and distal forearm.[30] Deep and superficial venous drainage are based on the cephalic vein and paired venae comitantes, respectively. Medial and lateral antebrachial cutaneous nerves of the forearm supply cutaneous sensation to the radial and volar forearm skin.

Flap elevation

The radial artery perforator flap can be raised based on any suitable perforator in the distal row of septocutaneous perforators as a pedicled or free flap. A pedicled radial artery perforator fasciocutaneous or turnover adipofascial (fascia and subcutaneous tissue) flap can be rotated to cover defects of the wrist and hand as distal as the proximal phalanges.[31] The superficial radial nerve and deep fascia should be preserved in the flap elevation, if possible. Perforators are dissected along the lateral intermuscular septum and the radial

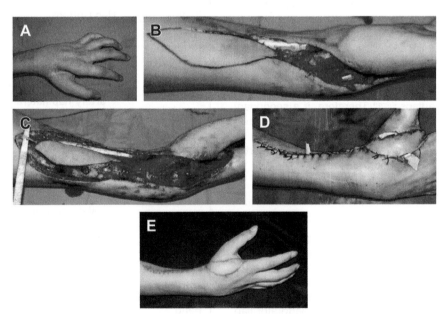

Fig. 4. Radial artery perforator flap. (*A*) A 21-year-old man with soft tissue defect dorsum hand, first web space, and a contracture deformity of first web space after injury. (*B*) Radial artery perforator flap was designed from the radial artery perforator. (*C*) Flap was elevated and the distal perforator pedicle was located 2 cm proximal to the radial styloid process. (*D*) Flap inset. Donor site closed primarily. (*E*) Follow-up. (*From* Yang D, Yang JF, Morris SF. Chapter 19: radial artery perforator flap. In: Blondeel PN, Morris SF, Hallock GG, et al, editors. Perforator flaps: anatomy, technique and clinical applications. 2nd edition. St. Louis (MO): Quality Medical Publishing; copyright 2013. p. 399; with permission.)

artery is then ligated proximally for a distally based pedicled flap transfer. A free radial artery perforator flap can be elevated with a very short segment of the radial artery (which can then be repaired primarily) and venous drainage provided by the cephalic vein.[32] Alternatively, a proximally based radial artery perforator flap may be elevated from the antebrachial surface of the forearm for coverage of the proximal forearm and elbow defects. For this flap variation, the skin paddle is designed at the middle third of the forearm with a pivot point located 5 cm from the interepicondylar line.[2,33] The distal perforators are ligated to increase the arc of rotation of the flap.[34]

Ulnar Artery Perforator Flap

The ulnar forearm fasciocutaneous flap is a favorable alterative to the radial forearm flap when thin, pliable, and sensate skin is desired for pedicled or free tissue transfer.[35,36] The ulnar forearm perforator flap has a more aesthetically pleasing, well-hidden donor site. It may be raised as a fasciocutaneous, functional myocutaneous (flexor carpi ulnaris), or osteomyocutaneous flap (ulna). Alternatively, the distally based dorsal ulnar artery perforator flap has the advantage of a longer vascular pedicle and avoids vascular damage to the dorsal ulnar nerve (**Fig. 5**).

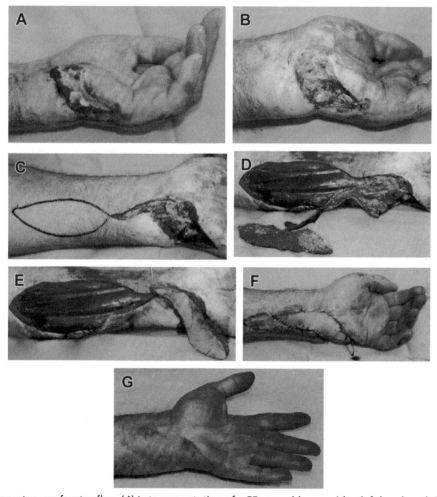

Fig. 5. Ulnar artery perforator flap. (*A*) Late presentation of a 55-year-old man with a left hand crush injury from an accident with an industrial ice machine. Full thickness wounds extending down to carpus with associated ulnar nerve and artery injuries. (*B*) Wound debridement and examination of ulnar nerve and artery. Ulnar nerve was damaged but intact. Ulnar artery was thrombosed over a span of 3 cm. (*C*) Ulnar artery perforator flap was designed on the most distal intact perforator of the ulnar artery. (*D, E*) Ulnar artery perforator flap elevation. (*F*) Flap inset. (*G*) The 6-month postoperative visit with slow recovery of ulnar nerve sensation. (*From* Yang D, Al Dhamin, Morris SF. Chapter 18: ulnar artery perforator flap. In: Blondeel PN, Morris SF, Hallock GG, et al, editors. Perforator flaps: anatomy, technique and clinical applications. 2nd edition. St. Louis (MO): Quality Medical Publishing; copyright 2013. p. 379; with permission.)

Vascular anatomy

The ulnar artery curves along the ulnar forearm giving off clusters of perforators along the ulnar aspect of the forearm. Most perforators are septo-cutaneous and are found within the fascial septum between flexor carpi ulnaris and the flexor digitorum superficialis muscle bellies.[37] The first perforator is reliably found 1 cm distal to the origin of the ulnar artery.[38] In a recent study, a perforator can be found within 3 cm and 6 cm diameter of the ulnar midpoint 94% and 100% of the time, respectively.[37]

At the wrist, the ulnar artery crosses the transverse carpal ligament on the radial side of the pisiform to form the superficial palmar arch. The dorsal branch of the ulnar artery originates 5 cm proximal to the pisiform in the forearm and runs distally along the flexor carpi ulnaris muscle trifurcating into ascending proximal, medial, and distal branches.[39] The distal branch of the dorsal ulnar artery runs alongside the dorsal branch of the ulnar nerve and courses distally to the proximal aspect of the abductor digiti minimi muscle where it anastomoses with branches from the deep ulnar artery.

Dual venous drainage is provided by a superficial (basilic vein) and deep venous system (paired venae comitantes). Cutaneous nerve supply is provided by the medial antebrachial cutaneous nerve, which travels adjacent to the basilic vein in the forearm. The median antebrachial nerve divides into an anterior branch to supply the anteromedial surface and an ulnar branch to supply the posterior medial surface of the forearm.

Flap elevation

The ulnar artery perforator flap is designed on the proximal or central forearm along a line between the medial epicondyle of the humerus to the lateral edge of the pisiform bone. Ninety-four percent of the time a large perforator is located within 3 cm of the midpoint of this line.[37] The cutaneous skin paddle is positioned on the proximal or distal forearm to take advantage of the cutaneous perforator clusters in those 2 locations.[40] Flap dissection is performed in a radial to ulnar and distal to proximal direction with the incorporation of the basilic vein. Septocutaneous perforators are identified and preserved along the intermuscular septum separating the flexor digitorum sublimis and the flexi carpi ulnaris muscles. If a sensate flap is desired, the anterior and ulnar branches of the medial antebrachial cutaneous nerves are identified and spared. The donor site is closed primarily or with a split-thickness skin graft.

The dorsal ulnar artery flap is a reliable option for the coverage of dorsal and volar wrist defects as well as distal hand defects.[37,41] The advantage of the dorsal ulnar artery flap is that it avoids sacrifice of a major arterial supply to the hand. This retrograde flap takes advantage of the anastomosis between the descending distal branch of the ulnar dorsal artery and the deep branch of the ulnar artery. The dorsal ulnar artery flap has a longer vascular pedicle as the ulnar dorsal artery is ligated at its origin in the forearm.

Posterior Interosseous Artery Flap

The posterior interosseous artery (PIOA) flap is a small- to moderate-sized fasciocutaneous flap that provides excellent color, texture, and size match for hand and wrist reconstruction.[2,42] More commonly raised as a reverse or free flap, the PIOA flap is used to cover defects of the distal wrist, hand, first web space, and proximal thumb.[43–45] The PIOA flap can be raised with a segment of radius as a vascularized bone graft.[43,46] The PIOA flap can be used to cover defects of the antecubital and volar forearm. A major advantage of this flap is that it does not require division or sacrifice of a major artery of the hand (**Fig. 6**).

Vascular anatomy

The PIOA arises from the common interosseous artery and infrequently from the ulnar artery in the proximal forearm and courses along the intramuscular septum between the extensor digiti minimi and the extensor carpi ulnaris muscles. In the proximal forearm, the PIOA runs deep alongside the posterior interosseous nerve. The PIOA emerges at the lower border of the supinator muscle and pierces the muscle belly of the abductor pollicis longus. In the distal forearm, the PIOA becomes superficial and travels on the extensor pollicis longus and extensor indicis muscles. The PIOA continues distally in the forearm to the proximal edge of the extensor retinaculum that corresponds to the pivot point for the reverse flap. Along the intermuscular septum, the PIOA gives off 4 to 7 septocutaneous perforators. In the middle third of the forearm, the PIOA consistently gives off a cutaneous perforator accompanied by 2 venae comitans that connect the superficial and deep venous systems of the flap.[47]

The PIOA anastomoses with the anterior interosseous artery (AIOA) 3 cm proximal to the distal radioulnar joint then extends to join the dorsal carpal arch. The anastomosis between the PIOA and AIOA can reliably be found 5 cm proximal to the ulnar styloid at the proximal edge of the pronator quadratus muscle. The AIOA/PIOA anastomosis is the basis of the distally based (reverse) PIOA flap. Venous drainage is provided by paired venae comitans that accompany the PIOA. Sensation to the PIOA flap is provided by the lower branch of

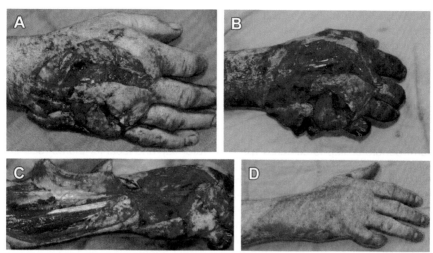

Fig. 6. PIOA flap. (*A*) 55-year-old man with significant soft tissue injury to dorsum right hand from a wood splitter accident involving comminuted fractures to long, ring, and little metacarpals. (*B*) Open reduction internal fixation of multiple metacarpal fractures using K wires. (*C*) Reverse PIOA perforator flap harvested based on the anterior interosseous perforating vessel. Split-thickness skin graft used to close donor site. (*D*) Six months postoperatively with residual flexion contracture of little finger.

the dorsal antebrachial and the medial antebrachial cutaneous nerves.

Flap elevation

The standard PIOA flap is centered on a line between the lateral epicondyle to the Distal radioulnar joint within the mid-forearm between the radial and ulna bones. Flap dissection occurs in a radial to ulnar and distal to proximal direction. Septocutaneous perforators are identified along the intermuscular septum. The middle septocutaneous perforator should be included within the flap because it contains the communicating vein between the superficial and deep venous system of the forearm and will improve venous drainage. Alternatively, a cutaneous vein should be incorporated into the flap for venous supercharging because venous congestion is not an uncommon complication of this flap.[47] The AIOA/PIOA anastomosis branch and interosseous recurrent artery are ligated, and the PIOA pedicle is dissected proximally to its origin deep to the supinator muscle. The reverse PIOA flap is positioned more proximally in the middle third of the forearm.[43,47] The anastomosis between the AIOA and PIOA is identified in the distal forearm beneath the indicis proprius and is preserved. Care is taken to preserve all communicating branches to the dorsal carpal arch. The proximal PIOA is ligated and the flap is passed through a wide subcutaneous tunnel to cover defects in the distal wrist and hand. If there is any pressure on the pedicle, the tunnel should be released to avoid vascular compromise.

Lateral Arm Perforator Flap

The lateral arm perforator flap is a versatile and relatively small flap but is ideal for coverage of smaller upper extremity wounds.[2,48] The lateral arm perforator flap can be raised as a fasciocutaneous, adipofascial, free fascial, or osteocutaneous (humerus) flap. The lateral arm perforator flap has a reliable vascular pedicle and reasonable donor site that can usually be closed primary. If the flap is harvested wider than about 6 to 7 cm, the donor site usually requires a skin graft for closure and is generally aesthetically unacceptable. The lateral arm perforator flap does not eliminate a major arterial supply to the hand. Disadvantages of this perforator flap relate to the bulkiness of the flap and the donor site if skin grafting is required.

Vascular anatomy

The lateral arm flap is based on the intermuscular septal perforators from the posterior radial collateral artery (PRCA), one of 2 main branches of the profunda brachial artery in the middle upper arm. The PRCA originates in the radial groove of the humerus and courses along the lateral intermuscular septum of the upper arm. The PRCA gives off 4 to 5 septocutaneous perforators along its course.[49] The most consistent perforator can be found 9 cm proximal to the lateral epicondyle along the intermuscular septum.[50] The lateral arm flap may be extended into the proximal forearm based on the rich vascular plexus that extends distally from the PCRA. Deep venous drainage is provided by the paired venae comitans, and the cephalic vein drains the superficial venous system. Nerve supply is provided by the lower lateral cutaneous nerve of the arm, a branch of the radial nerve.

Flap elevation

The lateral arm perforator flap is centered along the lateral intermuscular septum of the upper arm containing the dominant PRCA pedicle. The skin paddle is designed along a line from the deltoid insertion to the lateral epicondyle of the humerus. If the distal suprafascial plexus in the proximal forearm is included, the lateral forearm flap may be extended up to 12 cm beyond the lateral epicondyle. A branch of the PCRA consistently supplies the humerus between 2 and 7 cm proximal to the lateral epicondyle that may be harvested as a vascularized bone graft.[51] The lower lateral cutaneous or posterior cutaneous nerve of the forearm can also be harvested within the flap and used as a vascularized nerve graft for use in hand reconstruction.

FDMA Flap

The FDMA flap is an intrinsic hand-based perforator flap and ideal for thumb reconstruction. The reversed FDMA island flap is useful to reconstruct distal finger defects, such as the finger pulp.[52–54] Vascularized tendon (extensor indicis proprius), nerve (dorsal sensory branch of radial nerve), or bone (metacarpal) can also be included as a composite flap.[55] An extended reverse dorsal metacarpal artery flap is also described and is useful for coverage of defects distal to the proximal interphalangeal joint (**Fig. 7**).[56]

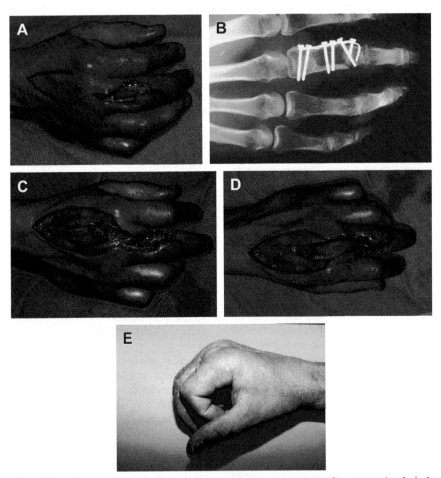

Fig. 7. FDMA flap. (*A*) A 26-year-old man with a gunshot wound to right long finger proximal phalanx with significant soft tissue and bone loss. (*B*) Open reduction and internal fixation with bone graft was performed to restore length and provide stable framework for soft tissue reconstruction. (*C*) Elevation of pedicled FDMA flap. The *X* marks perforator outlined intraoperatively by handheld Doppler probe. (*D*) Flap rotated 180° on pedicle and inset into defect. (*E*) Functional long-term recovery.

Vascular anatomy

The dorsal metacarpal arteries provide the vascular supply to the dorsal proximal portion of the hand. The deep palmar arch gives off dorsal perforating metacarpal arteries to supply the dorsal distal hand and proximal fingers. The FDMA originates from the radial artery and occasionally from the dorsal superficial antebrachial artery.[57] The FDMA travels parallel to the dorsal surface of the second metacarpal and superficial to the first dorsal interosseous muscle. At the level of the metacarpal neck, the FDMA anastomoses with dorsal perforating branches from the palmar metacarpal arteries. This anastomosis is the basis for the reverse FDMA flap.[52,58] The main cutaneous perforators are located just distal to the junctura tendinum and 1 cm proximal to the intermetacarpal head.[51] Venous drainage is provided by subcutaneous veins.

Flap elevation

The FDMA flap is dissected from distal to proximal by incising the most proximal edge of the flap over the dorsal aspect of the index finger proximal phalanx down to paratenon. The pivot point of the flap is determined by the location of the direct cutaneous perforator usually located 1 cm proximal to the intermetacarpal head and just distal to the junctura tendinum. The FDMA flap includes subcutaneous veins, the superficial radial nerve, and the first dorsal interosseous muscle fascia.[59] The flap is elevated with a cuff of fibrofatty tissue to avoid skeletonizing the pedicle. The reverse DMA flap, an extended version the FDMA, is possible by including the skin overlying the dorsum of the index finger.[60,61] For this flap, the pivot point is located distal to the metacarpophalangeal joint within the proximal third of the proximal phalanx so that the distal interphalangeal and palmar aspect of the finger pulp can be reached. The extended DMA flap is supplied by retrograde flow from first dorsal branch of the proper digital artery not the palmar perforator.

Propeller Flap

Perforator-based propeller flaps are island skin flaps with a propeller design that undergoes an axial rotation around its vascular pedicle to rotate up to 180° into an adjacent defect.[4] Several advantages of perforator-based propeller flaps exist. Propeller flaps provide an excellent color and texture match to cover an adjacent defect. A skeletonized perforator propeller flap allows for rotation without kinking the vascular pedicle. The propeller flap design provides a reliable and large-sized vascular pedicle to be located safely away from the zone of injury. Perforator-based

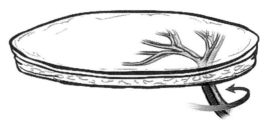

Fig. 8. Perforator-based propeller flap concept. (*From* Ogawa R, Hyakusoku H. Chapter 76: definition and nomenclature of propeller flaps. In: Blondeel PN, Morris SF, Hallock GG, et al, editors. Perforator flaps: anatomy, technique, and clinical applications. 2nd edition. St Louis (MO): Quality Medical Publishing; copyright 2013. p. 1309; with permission.)

propeller flaps have been used in traumatic lower extremity reconstruction with great success.[5,62] The same principles can be applied to traumatic upper extremity reconstruction because perforator-based propeller flaps can be designed anywhere a perforator is present (**Fig. 8**).[63,64] In the upper limb, perforator-based propeller flaps can be used to cover small- to medium-sized defects. For example, a radial collateral artery perforator-based propeller flap can be rotated for soft tissue coverage of small elbow defects less than 6 cm.[65] This particular flap for elbow coverage would be completed in a single-stage procedure and allow for early mobilization, which are 2 important principles of traumatic upper limb reconstruction.

SUMMARY

Perforator flaps are an excellent functional reconstruction option for complex upper extremity defects and add new tools to the toolbox of the reconstructive surgeon. Perforator flaps allow the transfer of like tissue into an adjacent defect in a single-stage procedure and for the optimization of an upper limb functional recovery. Our understanding of the cutaneous perforator anatomy has significantly evolved over the years and resulted in significant increase in the number of regional perforator flap options. An understanding of the upper extremity cutaneous perforator anatomy is essential for the design of local perforator flaps to reconstruct adjacent traumatic defects.

REFERENCES

1. Maciel-Miranda A, Morris SF, Hallock GG. Local flaps, including pedicled perforator flaps: anatomy, technique and applications. Plast Reconstr Surg 2013;131(6):896–911.

2. Sauerbier M, Unglaub F. Perforator flaps in the upper extremity. Clin Plast Surg 2010;37:667–76.

3. Hyakusoku H, Yamamoto T, Fumiiri M. The propeller flap method. Br J Plast Surg 1991;44(1):53–4.

4. Teo TC. The propeller flap concept. Clin Plast Surg 2010;37:615–26.

5. Gir P, Cheng A, Oni G, et al. Pedicled-perforator (propeller) flaps in lower extremity defects: a systemic review. J Reconstr Microsurg 2012;28(9): 595–601.

6. Georgescu AV, Matei I, Ardelean F, et al. Microsurgical nonmicrovascular flaps in forearm and hand reconstruction. Microsurgery 2007;27(5):384–94.

7. Kanellakos GW, Yang D, Morris SF. Cutaneous vasculature of the forearm. Ann Plast Surg 2003; 17:636–42.

8. Inoue Y, Taylor GI. Angiosomes of the forearm: anatomic study and clinical applications. Plast Reconstr Surg 1996;98:195–210.

9. Taylor GI, Palmer JH. The vascular territories (angiosomes) of the body: experimental study and clinical applications. Br J Plast Surg 1987;40(2): 113–41.

10. Taylor GI. Angiosome of the body and their supply to perforator flaps. Clin Plast Surg 2003;30(30): 331–42.

11. Saint-Cyr M, Wong C, Schaverien M, et al. The perforasome theory: vascular anatomy and clinical implications. Plast Reconstr Surg 2009;124:1529–44.

12. Taylor GI, Corlett RJ, Dhar SC, et al. The anatomical (angiosome) and clinical territories of cutaneous perforator arteries: development of the concept and designing safe flaps. Plast Reconstr Surg 2011;127(4):1447–59.

13. Rozen WM, Ashton MW, Le Roux CM, et al. The perforator angiosome: a new concept in design of deep inferior epigastric artery perforator flaps for breast reconstruction. Microsurgery 2010;30:1–7.

14. Taylor GI, Doyle M, McCarter G. Doppler probe for planning flaps: anatomic study and clinical applications. Br J Plast Surg 1990;43:1–16.

15. Schonauer F, Moio M, La Padula S, et al. Use of preoperative Doppler for distally based sural flap planning. Plast Reconstr Surg 2009;123:1639–40.

16. Lee GK. Invited discussion: harvesting of forearm perforator flaps based on intraoperative vascular exploration: clinical experiences and literature review. Microsurgery 2008;28:331–2.

17. Mathes SJ, Nahai MD. The reconstructive triangle: a Paradigm for surgical decision making. In: Mathes SJ, Nahai MD, editors. Reconstructive surgery: principles, anatomy & technique, Vol 1, 1st edition. New York: Churchill Livingstone; 1997. p. 9–36.

18. Morris SF, Gupta A, Saint-Cyr M. Chapter 55: flap options and technical considerations in the upper extremity. In: Blondeel PN, Morris SF, Hallock GG, et al, editors. Perforator flaps: anatomy, technique and clinical applications. 2nd edition. St Louis (MO): Quality Medical Publishing; 2013. p. 952–64.

19. Godina M. Early microsurgical reconstruction of complex trauma of the extremities. Plast Reconstr Surg 1986;78:285–92.

20. Lister G, Scheker L. Emergency free flap to the upper extremity. J Hand Surg Am 1988;13:22–8.

21. Harrison BL, Lakhiani C, Lee MR, et al. Timing of traumatic upper extremity free flap reconstruction: a systemic review and progress report. Plast Reconstr Surg 2013;132(3):591–6.

22. Serafin D, Shearin JC, Georgiade NG. The vascularization of free flaps: a clinical and experimental correlation. Plast Reconstr Surg 1977;60:233–41.

23. Tsur H, Daniller A, Strauch B. Neovascularization of skin flaps: route and timing. Plast Reconstr Surg 1980;66:85.

24. Coleman JJ III. Long-term evaluation of muscle and musculocutaneous flaps. In: Mathes SJ, Nahai F, editors. Clinical applications for muscle and musculocutaneous flaps. 1st edition. St Louis (MO): CV Mosby; 1982. p. 706–13.

25. Fisher L, Wood MB. Late necrosis of a latissimus dorsi free flap. Plast Reconstr Surg 1984;74:274.

26. Williams G, Butler P, Niranjan N. Flap vascularity after free flap musculocutaneous tissue transfer. Plast Reconstr Surg 1998;102:1781.

27. Ho AM, Chang J. Radial artery perforator flap. J Hand Surg 2010;35:308–11.

28. Herle M, Hafner HM, Dietz K, et al. Vascular dominance in the forearm. Plast Reconstr Surg 2003; 111:1891–8.

29. Saint-Cyr M, Mujadzic M, Wong C, et al. The radial artery pedicle perforator flap: vascular analysis and clinical implications. Plast Reconstr Surg 2010;125:2469–78.

30. Mateev MA, Ogawa R, Trunov L, et al. Shape-modified radial artery perforator flap method; analysis of 112 cases. Plast Reconstr Surg 2009; 123(5):1533–43.

31. Chang SM, Hou CL, Zang F, et al. Distally based radial forearm flap with preservation of radial artery: anatomic experimental and clinical studies. Microsurgery 2003;23:328–37.

32. Morris SF, Taylor GI. Predicting the survival of experimental skin flaps with the knowledge of the vascular architecture. Plast Reconstr Surg 1993; 92:1352–61.

33. Tiengo C, Macchi V, Porzionto A, et al. Anatomical study of perforator arteries in the distally based radial forearm fasciosubcutaneous flap. Clin Anat 2004;17:636–42.

34. Yang D, Morris SF, Tang M, et al. Reverse forearm island flap supplied by septocutaneous perforators of the radial artery: anatomic basis and clinical applications. Plast Reconstr Surg 2003;112(4): 1012–6.

35. Grobbelaar AO, Harrison DH. The distally based ulnar artery island flap in hand reconstruction. J Hand Surg Br 1997;22:204–11.

36. Koshima I, Lino T, Fukuda H, et al. The free ulnar forearm flap. Ann Plast Surg 1987;18:24–9.

37. Mathy JA, Moaveni Z, Tan ST. Perforator anatomy of the ulnar forearm fasciocutaneous flap. J Plast Reconstr Aesthet Surg 2012;65:1076–82.

38. El-Khatib HA, Mahboub TA, Ali TA. Use of an adipofascial flap based on the proximal perforators of the ulnar artery to correct contracture of elbow burn scars: an anatomic and clinical approach. Plast Reconstr Surg 2002;109:130–6.

39. Vergara-Amador E. Anatomical study of the ulnar dorsal artery and design of a new retrograde ulnar dorsal flap. Plast Reconstr Surg 2008;121(5): 1716–24.

40. Sun C, Hou ZD, Wang B, et al. An anatomic study on the characteristics of cutaneous branches-chain perforator flaps with ulnar artery pedicle. Plast Reconstr Surg 2013;131:329.

41. Beck C, Gilbert A. The ulnar flap- description and application. Eur J Plast Surg 1988;11:79–82.

42. Xu G, Lai-jin L. Coverage of skin defects in spaghetti wrist trauma: applications of the reverse posterior interosseous flap and its anatomy. J Trauma 2007;63:402–4.

43. Cheema TA, Lakshman S, Cheema MA, et al. Reverse-flow posterior interosseous flap: a review of 68 cases. Hand (N Y) 2007;2:112–6.

44. Agir H, Sen C, Alagoz S, et al. Distally based posterior interosseous flap: primary role in soft tissue reconstruction of the hand. Ann Plast Surg 2007; 59:291–6.

45. Ishiko T, Nakaima N, Suzuki S. Free posterior interosseous artery perforator flap for finger reconstruction. J Plast Reconstr Aesthet Surg 2009;62: e211–5.

46. Pagnotta A, Taglieri E, Molayem I, et al. Posterior interosseous artery distal radius graft for ulnar nonunion treatment. J Hand Surg Am 2012; 37(12):2605–10.

47. Shibata M. Posterior interosseous artery perforator flap. In: Blondeel PM, Hallock GG, Morris SF, et al, editors. Perforator flaps. St Louis (MO): Quality Medical Publishing; 2006. p. 270–82.

48. Akinci M, Ay S, Kamiloglu S, et al. Lateral arm free flaps in the defects of the upper extremity - a review of 72 cases. Hand Surg 2005;10(2–3):177–85.

49. Chen HC, el-Gammal TA. The lateral arm fascial free flap for resurfacing of the hand and fingers. Plast Reconstr Surg 1997;99(2):454–9.

50. Hwang K, Lee WJ, Jung CY, et al. Cutaneous perforators of the upper arm and clinical applications. J Reconstr Microsurg 2005;21(7):463–9.

51. Haas F, Rappi T, Koch H, et al. Free osteocutaneous lateral arm flap: anatomy and clinical applications. Microsurgery 2003;23(2):87–95.

52. Maruyama Y. Reverse dorsal metacarpal flap. Br J Plast Surg 1990;43(1):24–7.

53. Yang D, Morris SF. Reversed dorsal digital and metacarpal island flaps supplied by the dorsal cutaneous branches of the palmar digital artery. Ann Plast Surg 2001;46(4):444–9.

54. Dautel G, Merle M. Direct and reverse dorsal metacarpal flaps. Br J Plast Surg 1992;45(2):123–30.

55. Sherif MM. First dorsal metacarpal artery flap in hand reconstruction. I. Anatomical study. J Hand Surg Br 1995;19(1):26–31.

56. Shen H, Shen Z, Wang Y, et al. Extended reverse dorsal metacarpal artery flap for coverage of finger defects to the proximal interphalangeal joint. Ann Plast Surg 2013. [Epub ahead of print].

57. Foucher G, Braun JB. A new island flap transfer from the dorsum of the index to the thumb. Plast Reconstr Surg 1979;63(3):344–9.

58. Germann G, Hornung R, Raff T. Two new applications for the first dorsal metacarpal artery pedicle in the treatment of severe hand injuries. J Hand Surg Br 1995;20(4):525–8.

59. Small JO, Brennan MD. The first dorsal metacarpal artery neurovascular island flap. J Hand Surg Br 1988;13(2):136–45.

60. Gebhard B, Meissl G. An extended first dorsal metacarpal artery neurovascular island flap. J Hand Surg Br 1995;20(4):529–31.

61. Pelissier P, Cassoli V, Bakhach J, et al. Reverse dorsal digital and metacarpal flaps: a review of 27 cases. Plast Reconstr Surg 1999;103:159–65.

62. Pignatti M, Ogawa R, Hallock GG, et al. The "Tokyo" consensus on propeller flaps. Plast Reconstr Surg 2011;127:716–22.

63. Ono S, Sebastin SJ, Yazaki N, et al. Clinical applications of perforator based propeller flaps in upper limb soft tissue reconstruction. J Hand Surg Am 2011;36:853–63.

64. Lazzeri D, Huemer GM, Nicoli F, et al. Indications, outcomes, and complications of pedicled propeller perforator flaps for upper body defects: a systematic review. Arch Plast Surg 2013;40(1):44–51.

65. Murakami M, Ono S, Ishii N, et al. Reconstruction of elbow region defects using radial collateral artery perforator (RCAP)-based propeller flaps. J Plast Reconstr Aesthet Surg 2012;65(10):1418–21.

Local Flaps of the Hand

Shady A. Rehim, MB ChB, MSc, MRCS[a], Kevin C. Chung, MD, MS[b],*

KEYWORDS

- Hand flaps • Soft tissue coverage • Reconstruction

KEY POINTS

- When indicated, local hand flaps offer excellent coverage of soft tissue defects that replaces like with like.
- A variety of traditional and nontraditional local hand flaps can be used to cover most of small to moderate-sized defects of the hand.
- Although routinely used, the application of local hand flaps is an evolving field with multiple new flap designs and modifications being described based on the intricate vascular anatomy of the hand.
- Local hand flaps frequently result in optimum functional and aesthetic outcomes and may spare patients and surgeons from more complicated methods of soft tissue repair.

INTRODUCTION

The hand is an intricate part of the body that plays an essential role in social functioning, expression, productivity, and interactions with the environment.[1] The skin/soft tissue envelope of the hand is a complex structure that not only covers the underlying structures but also has specialized functional and sensory components. The thick glabrous skin of the palm withstands shearing forces encountered during daily activities and provides discriminatory sensory function that transfers touch, pain, and temperature, whereas the dorsal skin is pliable and mobile, and permits a wide range of motion of the hand such as finger pinch and grip.[1,2] Soft tissue defects of the hand following trauma or tumor resection are frequently encountered in hand surgery and may result in a temporary or permanent disability if not managed appropriately.

Over the past decades, several reconstructive procedures and their modifications have evolved to provide the ideal soft tissue coverage of the hand.[3] Conventionally, these included a range of options of primary wounds closure, skin grafts, local flaps, distant flaps, and micro-vascular free tissue transfer.[3–6] However, selecting the most suitable type of soft tissue cover for a particular defect can be a challenging process. Furthermore, the abundance of currently available reconstructive techniques makes this task difficult, especially for the inexperienced surgeon. When choosing one reconstructive method over another, it is prudent for the surgeon to have a sound knowledge of all available options, their limitations, complications, and expected outcomes. Reconstruction algorithms such as the reconstructive ladder, reconstructive elevator, and reconstructive matrix have been devised to assist surgeons in

Disclosure: None of the authors has a financial interest in any of the products, devices, or drugs mentioned in this article. This work was supported in part by grants from the National Institute of Arthritis and Musculoskeletal and Skin Diseases, National Institute on Aging (R01 AR062066), the National Institute of Arthritis and Musculoskeletal and Skin Diseases (2R01 AR047328-06), and a Midcareer Investigator Award in patient-oriented research (K24 AR053120) (K.C. Chung).

[a] Section of Plastic Surgery, Department of Surgery, University of Michigan Health System, 1500 East Medical Center Drive, Ann Arbor, MI 48109-5340, USA; [b] Section of Plastic Surgery, University of Michigan Medical School, University of Michigan Health System, 2130 Taubman Center, SPC 5340, 1500 East Medical Center Drive, Ann Arbor, MI 48109-5340, USA
* Corresponding author.
E-mail address: kecchung@med.umich.edu

Hand Clin 30 (2014) 137–151
http://dx.doi.org/10.1016/j.hcl.2013.12.004
0749-0712/14/$ – see front matter © 2014 Elsevier Inc. All rights reserved.

determining the most appropriate type of soft tissue reconstruction.[7,8] Although sometimes useful, there is no simple schema for reconstruction because every injury is different and every patient has a unique set of medical conditions. This article is a practical guide that offers an overview of several types of local hand flaps. With these flaps, most small-to-medium sized defects of the fingers, thumb, and dorsum of the hand can be reconstructed with minimal donor site morbidity and excellent functional and aesthetic results because a tissue defect is replaced with similar tissue type from its immediate anatomic vicinity.

GENERAL CONSIDERATIONS

A careful patient history and mechanism of the injury are indispensible in assessing the potential structural involvement and previous interventions. This provide a framework in which to begin treatment. One of the most influential factors in consideration of any treatment is tissue loss, including defect size, site, depth, orientation, and composition. However, other factors, such as those related to patients and surgeons' technical ability as well as the availability of resources, are of equal importance (**Table 1**). A systematic evaluation of all these factors is essential to individualize the reconstruction plan to each patient.

When closure of skin defects of the hand cannot be achieved by simple methods such as

healing by secondary intention or primary closure, other methods should be used. Skin grafts require a vascularized wound bed for the graft to take and are not suitable to cover defects over exposed tendons or bones without paratenon or periosteum. Furthermore, the high contracture potential, limited scar pliability, and poor sensibility limit their successful use as a primary method of reconstruction in the hand.[5] Locoregional or free tissue transfers bring their own blood supply, and thus have been frequently used to cover complex injuries with exposed tendons and bones. However, choosing between local flaps (harvested from adjacent tissue) or flaps (harvested from distant anatomic sites), several factors need to be considered. First, the simplest procedure that provides an adequate amount of tissue coverage and results in maximal gain of function together with the least amount of donor site deformity should be selected. Second, whenever possible, tissue replacement should follow the principle of replacing like with like to provide good color, texture, hairiness, and volume match.[8,9] Different regions of the hand have different functional and aesthetic requirements. For example, reconstructing highly sensate areas such as the fingertips with nonsensate skin may cripple the function of a patient's hand. In contrast, transposing skin containing hair follicles to a hairless surface such as the palm results in poor aesthetic appearance and patient dissatisfaction with surgery. Because of the special relationship between function and aesthetics of the hand, we have coined the term 'functional aesthetic units and subunits' of the hand by dividing the hand into distinct regions after taking into consideration the unique functional and aesthetic properties of each specific region that should be considered when planning for soft tissue reconstruction of the hand.

If there are no specific contraindications for local skin flaps such as crush injuries or the presence of local infection, they should be considered as the first line of treatment.[9] In addition to replacing like with like, the use of local skin flaps avoids the need for skin grafts or more extensive procedures such as free flaps. In all the following flap descriptions, we assume that other reconstructive options apart from local flaps have been weighed and rejected.

CLASSIFICATION OF SKIN FLAPS

A flap is skin with a varying amount of underlying tissue that is used to cover a defect and receives its blood supply from a source other than the tissue to which it is transferred to.[10,11] Skin flaps

Table 1 Perioperative considerations	
Wound	Size
	Site
	Side (eg, volar or dorsal)
	Amount and type of tissue loss (eg, isolated soft tissue injury or compound)
Donor site	Functional loss
	Scar location
	Morbidity
Flap	Texture
	Color
	Volume
	Hairiness
	Sensibility
Patient	Hand dominance
	Age
	Sex
	Occupation
	Medical comorbidities
	Preferences
Surgeon	Knowledge
	Technical skill
	Preference

can be classified according to their method of transfer (eg, advancement, rotation, and transposition),[11] composition (eg, cutaneous, fasciocutaneous, fascial, adipofascial, or compound flaps including bone and/or tendon),[12] and geometric design (eg, rhomboid, bilobed). If classified according to their location in relation to the defect alone, they can be grouped into 3 types of flaps[9]:

- Local flaps: harvested from the injured digit or tissue surrounding the injured zone of the hand
- Regional flaps: harvested from adjacent non-injured digit or zone of the hand
- Distant flaps: harvested away from the injured hand

If local skin flaps are further divided according to their blood supply, they can be grouped into random or axial pattern flaps as shown by McGregor in 1972.[13,14]

Random Pattern Flaps

Random pattern flaps have no known feeding blood vessel. Instead they are supplied by a random pattern of subdermal plexus and hence the name random pattern flaps. Because they lack a known vascular pedicle, the flap size is usually limited to a length/width ratio of 1:1 because of the limits of the perfusion pressure. However, this general rule does not strictly apply in highly vascularized areas such as the face or hands, in which a flap can be carefully extended to increase the flap length with respect to width in these areas. Examples of random pattern skin flaps include rotation, rhomboid, and transposition flaps.

Axial Pattern Flaps

Axial pattern flaps are based on a known artery that directly supplies a specific skin territory. Interconnections between branches of adjacent axial vessels exist that connect neighboring skin territories. Behan and Wilson were first to describe a system of linked axial pattern flaps via vascular communications based on a known arterial supply that was termed an angiotome.[15] Taylor and Palmer[16] later emphasized the role of these interconnections (choke vessels) and stated that when a flap is based on vessels of one angiosome, the corresponding tissue of adjacent angiosome can be safely captured based on the blood supply of the first angiosome.[17] Thus, in contrast with random pattern flaps, axial flaps may be extended beyond the 1:1 ratio to cover larger defects owing to their more robust blood supply because the axial vessel provides a larger perfusion territory.

An axial pattern flap can also be traced along its vascular pedicle thus converted to an island pedicled flap, which permits a greater freedom of mobility and increases the span of the flap to reach more distant defects. Although this can sometimes be advantageous, kinking or avulsion of the vascular pedicle jeopardizes the viability of the flap. Examples of axial pattern flaps include thumb neurovascular advancement flap (Moberg), first dorsal metacarpal artery flap, and second dorsal metacarpal artery flaps.

DORSUM OF THE HAND

Random pattern flaps such as rotation or transposition flaps are useful local skin flaps for coverage of a variety of soft tissue defects over the dorsal surface of the hand. By taking advantage of the skin laxity together with carefully measured geometric flap designs, clinicians can successfully move tissue around to close several skin defects. Furthermore, if used correctly, random pattern flaps can be applied throughout the hand and fingers. As a rule, clinicians should always perform a finger pinch test to decide which adjacent area provides most soft tissue for closure with respect to relaxed skin tension lines when executing these flaps so the donor site can be closed directly.

THE ROTATION FLAP

The name rotation flap refers to the vector of movement of the flap, which is usually curved or rotational. This flap can be thought of as the closure of a triangular defect by rotating adjacent skin around a rotation point (or fulcrum) into the defect (**Fig. 1**).[18] After outlining the defect, the arc of the flap rotation should be designed at least 3 to 4 times larger than the diameter of the defect to allow sufficient rotation of the flap and closure without excessive tension. A common mistake is to design a flap that is too small and cannot be sufficiently rotated into the defect. In these instances a small back cut or creation of a Burow triangle can help gain extra rotation. However, despite these maneuvers, the flap frequently cannot be sufficiently mobilized and creates a secondary defect from the donor site. Extending the back cut in order to gain further length may jeopardize the viability of the flap as it cuts through the blood supply at the base of the flap. It is therefore advisable to design a large flap from the outset to avoid this situation.

THE RHOMBOID/LIMBERG FLAP

First described by Limberg in 1928, the rhomboid flap is a transposition flap that consists of an equilateral parallelogram with 2 angles of 120° and 2 of

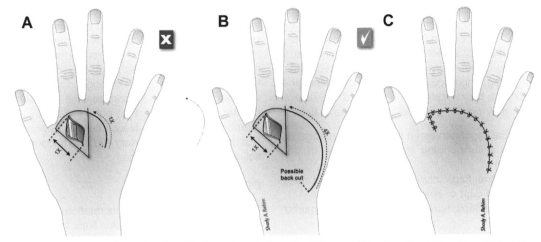

Fig. 1. Wrong design of rotation flap (*A*). Note that the length of the arc of the flap should be at least 3 to 4 times the diameter of the defect (*B*) to sufficiently rotate the skin flap into the defect (*C*).

60°.[19] To execute this flap, first the defect is converted into a rhomboid. A line is extended that equals the height of the rhomboid. This line is then extended parallel to one side of the rhomboid (**Fig. 2**A). The flap is elevated and transposed into defect, whereas the secondary defect is closed directly. In practice, defects have different sizes, shapes, and orientation. Strictly adhering to the measurements/angles described earlier may not provide the best aesthetic appearance. As the surgeon gains cumulative experience with performing these flaps, the flap design can be modified to better fit the defect. For example, the margins of the defect as well as the transposed skin of the rhomboid flap can be rounded/curved in a similar fashion to the bilobed flap. This maneuver eliminates the pointed triangular edges of the flap that

can be strangulated by tight skin closure during flap inset (see **Fig. 2**B). Furthermore, when designing the rhomboid flap on the dorsum of the hand, clinicians must be mindful that the line of closure of the secondary defect lies parallel to relaxed skin tension lines to avoid puckering of the skin and achieve skin closure without excessive tension.

FINGERS

It is easier to consider reconstruction of finger injuries if the fingers are divided into 3 parts: distal to the proximal interphalangeal (PIP) joint, at the level of PIP joint, and proximal phalanx. In addition to the level of injury, the side of injury should also be considered. Defects over palmar and dorsal

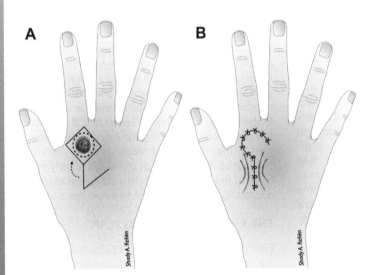

Fig. 2. A skin lesion (basal cell carcinoma) on the dorsum of the hand (*A*) and an outline of rhomboid flap planned for coverage of postexcision skin defect. Note that the line of flap closure should lie within the relaxed skin tension lines to facilitate skin closure taking advantage of the skin laxity (*B*). Also note that the margins of the transposed flap have been curved or rounded off to avoid strangulation and necrosis of pointed triangular edges of the skin flap.

surfaces of the fingers require different reconstruction options, as follows.

THE V-Y ADVANCEMENT FLAP

The V-Y advancement flap was first described by Tranquilli-Laeli in 1935 but was popularized by Atasoy and colleagues[20] in the United States in 1970.[21] Fingertip amputation is a common injury that frequently results in soft tissue defects with an exposed underlying bone of the distal phalanx that cannot be left to heal with secondary intention or covered by skin grafts. The availability of remaining adjacent soft tissue and the pattern of injury usually dictate the method of treatment. The V-Y advancement flap is most suitable for coverage of transverse or dorsal oblique fingertip amputations with exposed bone and sufficient nail bed support and length.[22] In addition, the V-Y advancement flap can be used to resurface adherent sensitive scars over fingertips resulting from previous amputation injuries. This flap provides excellent soft tissue replacement in terms of skin color, texture, sensation, and padding. However, in volar oblique fingertip amputations other options should be considered.

The V-Y advancement flap incorporates the volar digital neurovascular bundles that provide vascular and sensory supply to the flap. The first step of executing this flap includes marking the boundaries of the V-Y flap by drawing an inverted V on the volar side of the distal phalanx (**Fig. 3**A). The apex of the flap extends proximal toward the level of the distal interphalangeal (DIP) joint crease and the base extends distally to the radial and ulnar borders of the amputated nail bed. Extension of the skin incision beyond the DIP joint flexural

crease should be avoided because this may result in the development of skin contracture and flexion deformity of the distal phalanx. In contrast, extending skin incisions laterally beyond the borders of the nail bed may result in a flattened appearance of the nail bed. A combination of sharp and microscissors dissection is used to raise the flap. On either ends of the base of the flap, full-thickness skin incisions are performed that extend down to the periosteum to free periosteal attachments of the flap while preserving nourishing digital vessels. Toward the center, the flap is dissected off the flexor tendon sheath by carefully passing the tip and body of the scalpel from distal to proximal to the deep margin of the flap to cut through fibrofatty subcutaneous tissue to aid mobilization of the flap (see **Fig. 3**A). Once the flap is freed from its attachments, a skin hook is used to gently pull the distal end and advance the flap into the defect (see **Fig. 3**B, C). At this point, it should be emphasized that most of published textbook illustrations of the V-Y flap give the impression that the flap can easily be advanced forward. However, V-Y advancement flap has a limited mobility and only about 0.5 to 1 cm of advancement can be obtained, which limits the use of this flap to small fingertip defects. After flap advancement, the proximal wound is closed as a Y, hence the name V-Y advancement flap. The tourniquet is released to check perfusion of the flap and the distal end is sutured without excessive tension (**Fig. 4**).

THE THENAR FLAP

Gatewood[23] first described the technique of a thenar flap for coverage of fingertip injuries in

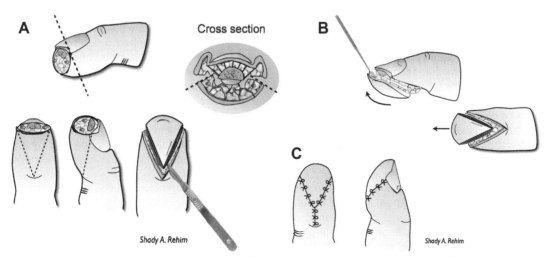

Fig. 3. Design of V-Y advancement flap to cover fingertip amputation (*A*). Note that the flap is outlined and dissected off flexor tendon sheath incorporating digital vessels and then advanced to cover the defect (*B, C*).

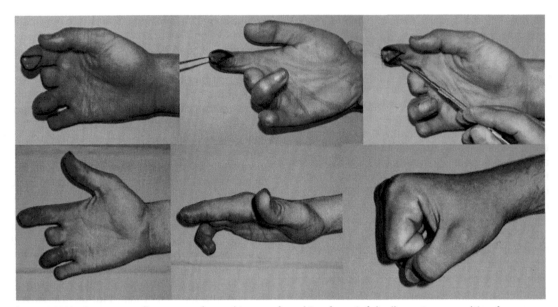

Fig. 4. A V-Y advancement flap was performed to resurface skin of a painful adherent scar resulting from a previous fingertip amputation of the index finger (*top*). Excellent soft tissue padding, contour, color, texture match, and mobility 9 months after surgery (*below*).

1926. This description was expanded on by Flatt[24,25] in 1957. The thenar flap is indicated for volar skin avulsions over the pulp of the finger (eg, volar oblique amputations); however, its use can also be extended to cover dorsal defects over the nail bed. Advantages of the thenar flap include inconspicuous donor site defect and good soft tissue padding, color, and texture match from the glabrous skin over the thenar area to the pulp of the finger. The major disadvantage of this flap is the propensity of PIP joint contracture and finger stiffness. Young women and children tend to have more supple joints and are therefore good candidates for the thenar flap.

The location of the donor site is identified by gently flexing the fingers toward the thenar eminence. The area of contact between the finger pulp and thenar eminence is the correct location of the donor site, which because of individual variation usually lies at or just proximal to the level of thumb metacarpophalangeal (MCP) joint. Excessive flexion of the finger results in marking a donor site too proximal on the palm, which eventually results in excessive tension on the flap and may jeopardize the success of the procedure. Once the correct donor site is identified, a rhomboid-shaped flap is designed; alternatively a circular or an H-shaped flap can be designed based on the shape and size of the finger defect (**Figs. 5 and 6**). The flap should be made slightly larger than the size of the defect. A full-thickness skin flap is then raised at the level of thenar muscle

fascia. Care must be taken not to injure the radial digital nerve of the thumb, which usually lies anterior to the midaxial lines of the thumb. Once the flap is elevated, the injured finger is advanced into the raw area to encompass the distal pulp space. The end of the flap is sutured to the defect and the donor site is closed primarily. The tourniquet is released to check the flap viability. The finger is left attached and after 2 to 3 weeks the flap is divided, thus replacing the original soft tissue defect with glabrous matching skin.

THE CROSS-FINGER FLAP

The cross-finger flap is a 2-staged flap reconstruction that was first described by Cronin[26] in 1951. Volar soft tissue defects located on the middle or distal phalanx can be covered with this flap. Another indication of the cross-finger flap is for more distal defects in which more tissue is required for coverage than can be obtained from a local advancement flap such as V-Y flap. Akin to thenar flap, PIP joint stiffness caused by joint flexion and immobilization is a concern when using the cross-finger flap.

The middle finger can be used to repair defects on either adjacent index or ring fingers, otherwise the donor finger is the one radial to the injured finger. The flap is outlined and elevated in an open book fashion in which a 3-sided rectangular or a rhomboidal flap is outlined on the dorsum of the middle phalanx of the healthy digit. The fourth

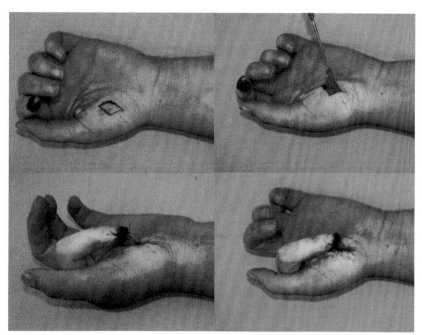

Fig. 5. A 20-year-old female patient who sustained a crush injury to the left index finger with soft tissue loss and necrosis. The necrotic skin was debrided, and a thenar flap was then designed to cover the open area.

side of the rectangular flap acts as the hinge of the flap located at the midaxial line of the finger nearest to the injured digit. A pattern can be used and transposed onto the donor site to estimate the size of the flap required. The flap should be designed slightly larger than the defect to avoid closure with excessive tension. A full-thickness skin flap is then raised over the paratenon of the underlying extensor tendon (**Figs. 7** and **8**). Care must be taken not to strip off the paratenon so that the secondary defect can be closed with a skin graft. After flap elevation, the flap is rotated 180° around its hinge and secured over the palmar defect of the adjacent injured finger. A full-thickness skin graft is then harvested to close the secondary defect. A Kirschner wire can be used to stabilize the fingers together to avoid pulling or detachment of

the flap, but this is not necessary in the authors' experience. The fingers are immobilized for approximately 2 to 3 weeks, after which a secondary procedure is performed to divide the skin bridge.

Pakian[27] first used a modification of the cross-finger flap known as the reverse cross-finger flap for defects located on the dorsal side of the fingers. In principle, the reverse cross-finger flap is similar to the classic cross-finger flap; however, the technique is slightly different. The flap is designed within the functional limits of the phalanx on the dorsal aspect of the adjacent noninjured finger. A cross-finger flap should not be harvested from the volar side of the finger because this leads to volar scar contracture and leaves a major donor site problem. The same open-book technique of raising a 3-sided rectangle with the fourth side

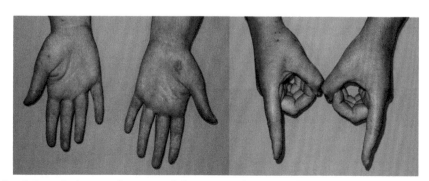

Fig. 6. Results of the soft tissue replacement of the same patient as in **Fig. 4** 2 months after surgery.

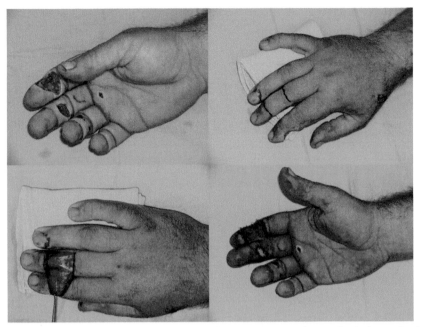

Fig. 7. A 49-year-old who had an electric burn injury with entrance wound over the index and middle fingers. Following wound debridement the patient had an exposed flexor tendon that was covered with a cross-finger flap obtained from the dorsum of the middle phalanx of the adjacent long finger.

acting as a hinge adjacent to the injured finger is used. The skin is raised at the level of the deep dermis leaving behind the rest of the deep layer of dermis and subcutaneous tissue, which in turn is raised in the same manner over the paratenon

and reflected 180° to cover the primary defect. By doing so, the superficial surface of the subcutaneous flap lies directly on the wound bed of the primary defect, and its deep surface becomes superficial and is subsequently covered with a

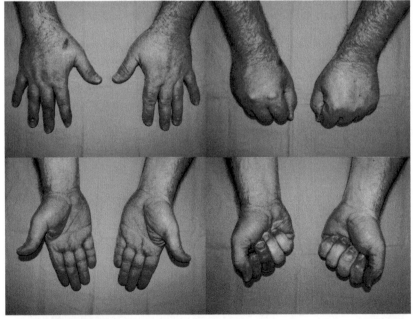

Fig. 8. Results of soft tissue replacement with cross-finger flap of the same patient as in **Fig. 6** 5 months after surgery.

full-thickness skin graft (**Fig. 9**). The skin flap that was initially raised from the donor site is then reflected back to cover the secondary defect. After a period of 2 to 3 weeks the bridge of the subcutaneous flap can be safely divided.

THE HOMODIGITAL ISLAND FLAP

Weeks and Wray[28] in 1973 described the homodigital island flap that is based on the volar blood supply of the fingers, either the radial or ulnar digital artery and its venae comitantes. The flap can be harvested on a proximal (antegrade) or a distal (retrograde) pedicle.[29] Proximally based flaps are used to cover more proximal defects, whereas reverse pedicle digital island flaps, described by Lai and colleagues,[30] are used to cover more distal defects over PIP and DIP joints (**Fig. 10**). In contrast with the cross-finger flap, the advantages of this flap include that it is a single-stage

procedure confined to the injured digit. However, hand surgeons are currently less enthusiastic to perform this flap because of fine dissections and increased risk of damage of the vascular pedicle as well as decrease of sensation over the donor site, especially in dominant fingers. Furthermore, this flap is not suitable for patients with peripheral vascular disease or in digits nourished by a single vessel. A positive digital Allen test showing incomplete collateral perfusion is therefore a contraindication to the use of this flap.[21]

For the reverse pedicle digital island flap, the flap is outlined on the lateral border of the base of the affected digit. A pattern is used and transferred onto the donor area to estimate the size of the flap required. In general, the flap should be designed slightly larger than the defect to allow for primary skin contraction. Dissection is performed from proximal to distal until enough length of the pedicle is obtained, which usually corresponds

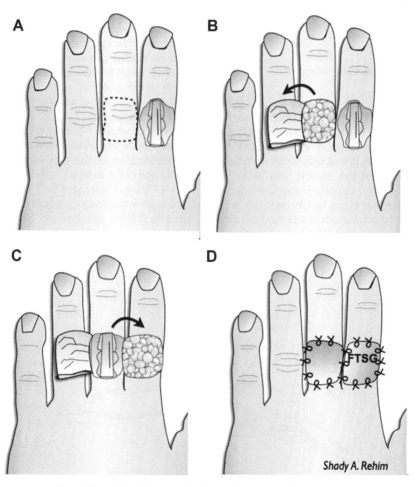

Shady A. Rehim

Fig. 9. The reverse cross-finger flap. The skin over the donor finger is reflected leaving part of the deep dermis and subcutaneous tissue (*A, B*) that is in turn swung over the primary defect and covered with a full-thickness skin graft. Reflecting back the skin that was initially elevated closes the secondary defect created over the donor finger (*C, D*).

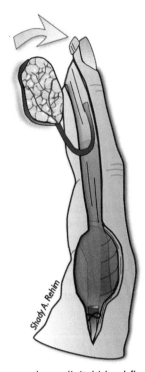

Fig. 10. A reverse homodigital island flap.

with the level of the DIP joint. During dissection the digital nerve is gently separated from the vascular pedicle and the digital vessel is ligated proximally. The pedicle should be raised with a cuff of fat; attempts to skeletonize the pedicle may result in damage of the venous drainage or vascular supply of the flap. Once the island flap is elevated, it is rotated into the defect and sutured loosely to avoid compression of the pedicle. A full-thickness skin graft is then harvested to close the secondary defect.

THE DORSAL METACARPAL ARTERY FLAP

In 1987, Earley and Milner[31] first described the proximally based dorsal metacarpal artery flap based on the first and second dorsal metacarpal artery. In 1990, Quaba and Davison[32] introduced another subset of flaps called the distally based dorsal metacarpal artery (DMCA) flap, which is not based on the dorsal metacarpal arteries but on a constant palmar-dorsal perforator present in the digital web space (**Fig. 11**). The DMCA flap became a popular flap for coverage of dorsal finger defects up to the level of the PIP joint. Several flap modifications have since been devised based on the vascular anatomy of the DMCA and the more distal dorsopalmar digital cutaneous perforators in order to increase the span of the flap to reach more distal defects.[33–37]

The DMCA flap is indicated for large dorsal finger defects or when a 1-stage procedure is preferred to allow finger mobilization. The flap can also be used to reconstruct volar defects over the proximal; however, this should be discouraged because the transposition of hairy pigmented skin from the dorsal surface of the hand is not an ideal match to the glabrous, lighter-colored skin of the palmar surface of the fingers, especially in dark-skinned individuals.

The flap is usually centered on the location of the palmar-dorsal perforator of the deep palmar arch. The boundaries of the flap extend between the distal edge of the extensor retinaculum proximally, the MCP joint distally, and the outer borders of the adjoining metacarpals on either side.[38] The flap is harvested from proximal to distal, raising the skin flap above the paratenon of the underlying extensor tendon. The pedicle is traced along the course of the perforator that usually arises

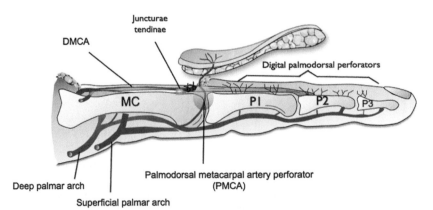

Fig. 11. The vascular supply of the distally based DMCA perforator flap as described by Quaba and Davidson. (*Data from* Quaba AA, Davison PM. The distally-based dorsal hand flap. Br J Plast Surg 1990;43(1):28–39.)

immediately distal to the juncturae tendinum at the interdigital space. There should be no attempt to isolate the perforator because this may lead to its damage and affect flap viability. At this point the tourniquet is released to check flap perfusion. The flap is then rotated and passed through a subcutaneous tunnel to reach the defect (**Figs. 12** and **13**). The primary defect is closed by primary closure and the fingers and wrist are immobilized in extension.

The DMCA flap can be modified to reach more distant defects over the dorsum of the middle/distal phalanx. This modification may involve designing the flap as a curved ellipse instead of a straight ellipse. After raising the flap, straightening the curved skin ellipse during flap inset offers an additional 8 to 10 mm of length (**Fig. 14**). Another maneuver involves dividing and ligating the DMCA proximal to the perforator. Because a perforator arising from the deep palmar arch directly nourishes this flap, its attachment with the DMCA can be carefully divided to allow a greater advancement of the flap.[38]

THUMB

The thumb represents 40% to 50% of hand function.[39] Restoring thumb defects is essential for pulp-to-pulp and key pinch grip. The arterial supply of the thumb differs from that of other fingers. The volar side of the thumb is supplied by 2 palmar collateral arteries arising from the princeps pollicis artery, which in turn is derived from the radial artery at the first intermetacarpal web space.[40] The dorsal blood supply of the thumb is independent from its volar circulation. The skin over the dorsum of the thumb is predominantly supplied by ulnar dorsocollateral and radial dorsocollateral arteries, which are branches of the radial artery. Based on knowledge of the anatomic blood supply of the thumb, several local flaps can be elevated to reconstruct volar and dorsal defects, as follows.

THE MOBERG FLAP

The advancement neurovascular flap of the thumb was originally described by the Erik Moberg[41] in 1964 hence it is best known today as the Moberg flap. The Moberg flap is indicated for coverage of small-to-medium sized defects over the volar aspect of the distal phalanx of the thumb without the need to shorten the length. This flap provides excellent soft tissue coverage with highly sensate, well-padded skin of similar color and texture. The main disadvantage of the Moberg flap is the tendency for interphalangeal (IP) joint flexion deformity if the flap is insufficiently mobilized to cover the volar distal defect.

The flap is outlined along midaxial lines on either sides of the thumb. The proximal border of the flap should correspond with the level of flexural crease of the MCP joint. At the distal end of the flap, a full-thickness skin incision is made along the midaxial lines. Care must be taken not to sever the neurovascular bundles nourishing the flap that lie just anterior to the midaxial crease (**Fig. 15**). The flap is gently dissected off the flexor pollicis longus tendon incorporating digital vessels and nerves. Once the flap is freed from all but its proximal attachment, the flap can be advanced 1 to 1.5 cm toward the distal end and sutured to the tip of the thumb to cover the defect without excessive tension. Often the flap cannot be advanced enough to cover the defect. In these instances minimal trimming of the distal phalanx can be performed. As an alternative, the IP joint can be slightly flexed. However, in order to preserve the length of the thumb and prevent flexion deformity of the IP joint, the proximal end of the flap can be modified to extend across the MCP flexural crease as a V-shaped incision, converting the flap into an island flap to gain further length. After advancing the flap the proximal wound is closed in a V-Y fashion. Another type of flap modification involves making a proximal transverse incision along the MCP joint crease; again, this converts the flap into an island flap. However, the resultant skin defect is not directly closed, and alternatively can be covered with a full-thickness skin graft to avoid the development of vertical skin contractures across the MCP joint. When executing these modifications, care is needed to preserve the

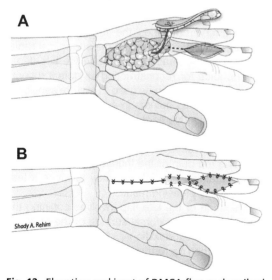

A

B

Shady A. Rehim

Fig. 12. Elevation and inset of DMCA flap as described by Quaba and Davidson[32] (*A*) to cover a defect over the dorsum of the finger (*B*).

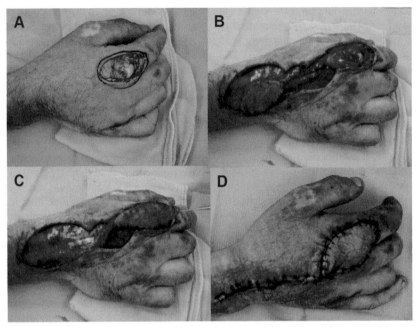

Fig. 13. A 34-year-old male patient who sustained a full-thickness electric burn injury over the dorsum of his left index finger. Following wound debridement a wound defect measuring 6 × 3 cm with an underlying exposed MCP joint was created (*A*). A DMCA flap was raised (*B*) then mobilized (*C*) to cover the wound (*D*).

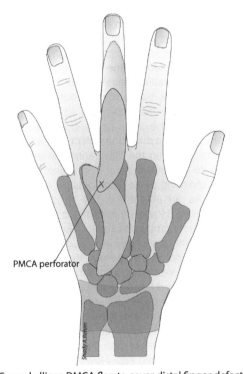

Curved ellipse DMCA flap to cover distal finger defects

Fig. 14. An ellipse design of the skin paddle of the DMCA flap that can be stretched owing to skin elasticity to reach more distant defects on dorsum of the finger. PMCA, palmar metacarpal artery.

neurovascular bundles, and these modifications should only be performed when necessary.

THE FIRST DMCA FLAP (KITE FLAP)

Foucher and Braun[42] in 1979 described the first DMCA flap, also known as the kite flap because the flap is raised with the pedicle, which resembles a kite. The kite flap is a skin island flap harvested from the dorsal surface of the adjacent index finger. The constant first DMCA, a branch of the radial artery, nourishes the flap. The flap may also incorporate a branch of the superficial radial nerve. These characteristics make the kite flap a good choice for reconstructing all dorsal defects of the thumb and can be used to restore sensibility over thumb pulp defects in a single-stage procedure. The disadvantages of this flap may include creating a conspicuous donor site defect that is closed with a skin graft. Furthermore, when reconstructing the pulp of the thumb, the darker dorsal skin containing hair follicles may produce a less aesthetically pleasing result.

Execution of the kite flap involves outlining the boundaries on the dorsal surface of the proximal phalanx of the index finger. A full-thickness skin incision is then performed and the flap is dissected from distal to proximal. The flap is elevated together with the underlying fascia of the first interosseus muscle incorporating the vascular pedicle that runs deep in the overlying fascial pocket.

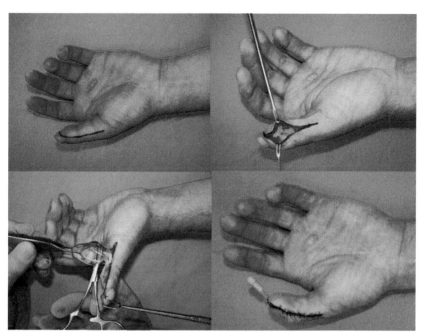

Fig. 15. A 22-year-old male patient who had a crush injury to the left thumb with loss of tissue at the nail bed that was treated initially with primary closure and left him with thin sensitive skin over the tip of the thumb. Following scar excision, a Moberg flap was performed to reconstruct the resultant defect. Note the digital nerves incorporated within the flap (*left bottom*).

The pedicle is harvested with a cuff of subcutaneous tissue and no effort should be made to identify or isolate the pedicle because this may damage its blood supply. The pedicle is then traced back to a point near its base at the anatomic snuff-box that contains the radial artery to allow rotation of the flap. Once the flap and the pedicle are dissected, the perfusion of the flap is checked by temporarily deflating the tourniquet. A subcutaneous tunnel is then created in order to place the flap through the tunnel and into the thumb defect. The subcutaneous tunnel must be spacious enough not to exert

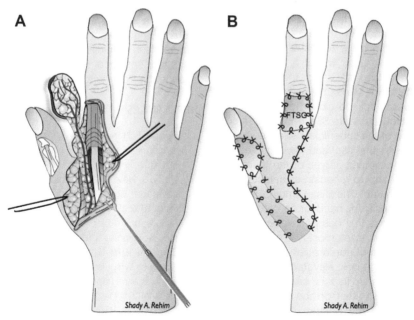

Fig. 16. Harvesting (*A*) and transfer (*B*) of the first dorsal metacarpal artery flap to cover dorsal thumb defect. FTSG, full-thickness skin graft.

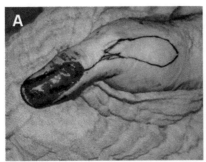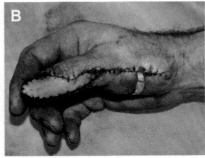

Fig. 17. A dorsoradial thumb defect (*A*) covered by reverse dorsoradial flap (Moschella flap) of the thumb (*B*). The dorsoulnar flap (Brunelli flap) is performed in a similar fashion but elevated from the dorsoulnar side of the thumb. (*From* Germann G, Bidermann N, Levin SL. Intrinsic flaps in the hand. Clin Plast Surg 2011;38(4):729–38; with permission.)

any pressure on the pedicle. As an alternative, a skin paddle is harvested over the pedicle that can be transposed along the path of the flap to the defect. We prefer this flap design to avoid passing the flap through the tunnel, which can kink the pedicle (**Fig. 16**). The donor defect is usually closed by a full-thickness graft.

THE DORSOULNAR AND DORSORADIAL COLLATERAL ARTERY FLAPS

The reverse flow homodigital dorsoulnar and dorsoradial collateral artery flaps (**Fig. 17**) were described by Brunelli (1993)[43–45] and Moschella and Cordova (2006),[46,47] respectively. These flaps are supplied by the ulnar dorsocollateral and radial dorsocollateral arteries, which arise from the radial artery at the level of the head of the first metacarpal bone and run on their respective sides to supply the skin over the dorsum of the thumb. Studies have shown the constancy of these vessels, but a Doppler examination helps to identify the course of the vessel and to mark the pivot point of the flap.[29] The advantage of using these flaps is 2-fold. First, the donor site is confined to the thumb and in most cases can be closed primarily, thus leaving inconspicuous scars. Second, the dorsocollateral branch of the superficial radial nerve can be harvested with the flap and reconnected to one of the volar collateral nerves of the thumb to create a sensate flap to reconstruct defects over the pulp of the thumb. The disadvantage associated with these flaps is the need for delicate micro-dissection, a process that has been described as microsurgery without anastomosis.

The dorsoulnar and dorsoradial reverse flow collateral artery flaps are elevated in a similar fashion. First, the skin flap is centered on the feeding blood vessel either on the dorsoulnar or dorsoradial sides of the dorsum of the thumb, based on the type of flap to be executed. Flap dissection is performed from proximal to distal to avoid damaging the pedicle. Clinicians should always avoid isolating the pedicle. Dissection of the flap is continued to a level at the middle of the proximal phalanx to preserve the anastomosis between palmar and dorsal vessels. At this point the tourniquet is deflated to check perfusion of the flap. The flap is then reflected and secured to the defect taking care not to compress the pedicle. A cutaneous tail should be harvested to avoid tunneling of the flap and to allow for primary skin closure after rotation of the flap into the defect.[47]

SUMMARY

If there are no clinical restrictions, local flaps represent an ideal soft tissue cover for small and moderate soft tissue defects. A surgeon who is well versed in the vascular anatomy of the hand and different types of local flap reconstruction is able to treat a variety of defects without requiring more complex methods of soft tissue repair. Nonetheless, clinicians must also recognize the limitations of local flaps and be prepared to change the treatment plan if the necessity arises.

REFERENCES

1. Hegge T, Henderson M, Amalfi A, et al. Scar contractures of the hand. Clin Plast Surg 2011;38(4):591–606.
2. Upton J, Havlik RJ, Khouri RK. Refinements in hand coverage with microvascular free flaps. Clin Plast Surg 1992;19(4):841–57.
3. McGregor IA. Flap reconstruction in hand surgery: the evolution of presently used methods. J Hand Surg Am 1979;4(1):1–10.
4. Rockwell WB, Lister GD. Soft tissue reconstruction. Coverage of hand injuries. Orthop Clin North Am 1993;24(3):411–24.
5. Giessler GA, Germann G. Soft tissue coverage in devastating hand injuries. Hand Clin 2003;19(1):63–71, vi.

6. Friedrich JB, Katolik LI, Vedder NB. Soft tissue reconstruction of the hand. J Hand Surg Am 2009; 34(6):1148–55.

7. Gottlieb LJ, Krieger LM. From the reconstructive ladder to the reconstructive elevator. Plast Reconstr Surg 1994;93(7):1503–4.

8. Maciel-Miranda A, Morris SF, Hallock GG. Local flaps, including pedicled perforator flaps: anatomy, technique, and applications. Plast Reconstr Surg 2013;131(6):896e–911e.

9. Foucher G, Boulas HJ, Braga Da Silva J. The use of flaps in the treatment of fingertip injuries. World J Surg 1991;15(4):458–62.

10. Pederson WC, Lister G. Local and regional flap coverage of the hand. In: Wolfe SW, editor. Green's operative hand surgery. 6th edition. Philadelphia: Elsevier Churchill Livingstone; 2011. p. 1662.

11. Lister G. Local flaps to the hand. Hand Clin 1985; 1(4):621–40.

12. Cormack GC, Lamberty BG. A classification of fasciocutaneous flaps according to their patterns of vascularisation. Br J Plast Surg 1984;37(1):80–7.

13. McGregor IA, Morgan G. Axial and random pattern flaps. Br J Plast Surg 1973;26(3):202–13.

14. McGregor IA, Jackson IT. The extended role of the deltopectoral flap. Br J Plast Surg 1970;23:173.

15. Lamberty BG, Cormack GC. Progress in flap surgery: greater anatomical understanding and increased sophistication in application. World J Surg 1990; 14(6):776–85.

16. Taylor GI, Palmer JH. The vascular territories (angiosomes) of the body: experimental study and clinical applications. Br J Plast Surg 1987;40(2):113–41.

17. Taylor GI. The angiosomes of the body and their supply to perforator flaps. Clin Plast Surg 2003; 30(3):331–42, v.

18. Birkbeck DP, Moy OJ. Anatomy of upper extremity skin flaps. Hand Clin 1997;13(2):175–87.

19. Chasmar LR. The versatile rhomboid (Limberg) flap. Can J Plast Surg 2007;15(2):67–71.

20. Atasoy E, Ioakimidis E, Kasdan ML, et al. Reconstruction of the amputated finger tip with a triangular volar flap. A new surgical procedure. J Bone Joint Surg Am 1970;52(5):921–6.

21. Chao JD, Huang JM, Wiedrich TA. Local hand flaps. J Hand Surg Am 2001;1(1):25–44.

22. Ramirez MA, Means KR Jr. Digital soft tissue trauma: a concise primer of soft tissue reconstruction of traumatic hand injuries. Iowa Orthop J 2011;31:110–20.

23. Gatewood A. A plastic repair of finger defects without hospitalization. JAMA 1926;87:1479.

24. Flatt AE. The thenar flap. J Bone Joint Surg Br 1957; 39(1):80–5.

25. Flatt AE. Minor hand injuries. J Bone Joint Surg 1955;37:117.

26. Cronin T. The cross finger flap: a new method of repair. Am Surg 1951;17:419–25.

27. Foucher G, Merle M, Debry R. The reversed de-epithelialized flap. Ann Chir Main 1982;1(4):355–7.

28. Weeks PM, Wray RC. Management of acute hand injury. St Louis (MO): Mosby; 1973.

29. Germann G, Biedermann N, Levin SL. Intrinsic flaps in the hand. Clin Plast Surg 2011;38(4):729–38.

30. Lai CS, Lin SD, Yang CC. The reverse digital artery flap for fingertip reconstruction. Ann Plast Surg 1989;22:495–500.

31. Earley MJ, Milner RH. Dorsal metacarpal flaps. Br J Plast Surg 1987;40(4):333–41.

32. Quaba AA, Davison PM. The distally-based dorsal hand flap. Br J Plast Surg 1990;43(1):28–39.

33. Maruyama Y. The reverse dorsal metacarpal flap. Br J Plast Surg 1990;43:24–7.

34. Pelissier P, Casoli V, Bakhach J, et al. Reverse dorsal digital and metacarpal flaps: a review of 27 cases. Plast Reconstr Surg 1999;103(1):159–65.

35. Bene MD, Petrolati M, Raimondi P, et al. Reverse dorsal digital island flap. Plast Reconstr Surg 1994;93:552.

36. Santa Comba A, Amarante J, Silva A, et al. Reverse dorsal metacarpal osteocutaneous flaps. Br J Plast Surg 1997;50(7):555–8.

37. Gregory H, Heitmann C, Germann G. The evolution and refinements of the distally based dorsal metacarpal artery (DMCA) flaps. J Plast Reconstr Aesthet Surg 2007;60(7):731–9.

38. Sebastin SJ, Mendoza RT, Chong AK, et al. Application of the dorsal metacarpal artery perforator flap for resurfacing soft-tissue defects proximal to the fingertip. Plast Reconstr Surg 2011;128(3):166e–78e.

39. Bunnell S. Reconstruction of the thumb. Am J Surg 1958;95(2):168–72.

40. Brunelli F, Vigasio A, Valenti P, et al. Arterial anatomy and clinical application of the dorsoulnar flap of the thumb. J Hand Surg Am 1999;24(4):803–11.

41. Moberg E. Aspects of sensation in reconstructive surgery of the upper extremity. J Bone Joint Surg Am 1964;46:817–25.

42. Foucher G, Braun JB. A new island flap transfer from the dorsum of the index to the thumb. Plast Reconstr Surg 1979;63(3):344–9.

43. Brunelli F. Le lambeau dorso-cubital du pouce. Ann Chir Main 1993;12:105–14.

44. Terán P, Carnero S, Miranda R, et al. Refinements in dorsoulnar flap of the thumb: 15 cases. J Hand Surg Am 2010;35(8):1356–9.

45. Moschella F, Cordova A, Pirrello R, et al. Anatomic basis for the dorsal radial flap of the thumb: clinical applications. Surg Radiol Anat 1996;18:179.

46. Moschella F, Cordova A. Reverse homodigital dorsal radial flap of the thumb. Plast Reconstr Surg 2006; 117(3):920–6.

47. Hrabowski M, Kloeters O, Germann G. Reverse homodigital dorsoradial flap for thumb soft tissue reconstruction: surgical technique. J Hand Surg Am 2010;35(4):659–62.

Flap Reconstruction of the Elbow and Forearm
A Case-Based Approach

Joshua M. Adkinson, MD[a], Kevin C. Chung, MD, MS[b],*

KEYWORDS

- Elbow wounds • Forearm wounds • Flap reconstruction

KEY POINTS

- Forearm wounds can generally be closed by recruitment of local tissues. Only wounds with exposed neurovascular structures, tendon, or bone typically require flap coverage.
- Elbow wounds frequently involve bone, joints, tendons, neurovascular structures, and prostheses; these factors, combined with the requirement for early motion, mandate a well-padded and durable flap reconstruction.
- A multitude of options exist for reconstructing elbow and forearm wounds.
- It is imperative to understand the indications, advantages, and disadvantages of each flap.

INTRODUCTION

Elbow and forearm wounds range from those caused by congenital anomalies, contracture release, tumor excision, and burns, to those caused by autoimmune disease, trauma, infection, and exposed prostheses.[1] Regardless of the cause, wounds about the elbow and forearm have potentially disabling effects,[2] influencing both the ability to work and quality of life. An appreciation for the origin and socioeconomic implications of upper extremity wounds is imperative for a successful outcome.

Elbow and forearm wounds require a stable and durable solution. Important differences remain, however, regarding the reconstructive demands intrinsic to each anatomic area. Forearm wounds can often be closed directly or covered with skin grafts. Only large wounds or those with exposed neurovascular structures, tendon, or bone typically require flap closure. Conversely, elbow wounds have limited simple solutions for coverage, because underlying structures and prostheses are easily exposed.[3] Elbow wounds also have the unique requirement of a pliable yet well-padded reconstruction. These characteristics promote early mobilization to prevent contracture and stiffness.[4] Because local tissues are frequently involved in the zone of injury or lack characteristics necessary to achieve an optimal outcome, the surgeon often must choose from the myriad of available flap options.

PRINCIPLES OF RECONSTRUCTION

The reconstructive ladder[5] is an important concept in wound management. Large, complex wounds of the forearm and many elbow wounds

---

Supported in part by grants from the National Institute on Aging and National Institute of Arthritis and Musculoskeletal and Skin Diseases (R01 AR062066) and from the National Institute of Arthritis and Musculoskeletal and Skin Diseases (2R01 AR047328-06) and a Midcareer Investigator Award in Patient-Oriented Research (K24 AR053120) (to K.C. Chung).

[a] Section of Plastic Surgery, Department of Surgery, University of Michigan Health System, 2130 Taubman Center, SPC 5340, 1500 East Medical Center Drive, Ann Arbor, MI 48109-5340, USA; [b] Section of Plastic Surgery, University of Michigan Medical School, 2130 Taubman Center, SPC 5340, 1500 East Medical Center Drive, Ann Arbor, MI 48109-5340, USA
* Corresponding author.
E-mail address: kecchung@med.umich.edu

Hand Clin 30 (2014) 153–163
http://dx.doi.org/10.1016/j.hcl.2013.12.005

may require initial management with local, regional, distant, or free flap coverage (reconstructive elevator) (**Fig. 1**).[1,6] Wound characteristics are important, including origin, size, orientation, and exposure of or injury to bone and neurovascular structures. Patient comorbidities, donor site availability, and clinical status also directly impact the options for flap closure. Previous trauma and surgery to the affected extremity are particularly relevant when considering local and regional flap coverage. The ulnar nerve should be carefully identified during any soft tissue reconstruction of the posterior or medial elbow. Because both debridement and flap elevation in this unique area put the nerve at risk, the surgeon should consider concomitant ulnar nerve transposition.[7]

Timing of definitive reconstruction can affect the ultimate outcome. Reconstruction must be delayed until contamination has been cleared, but should be early enough to facilitate therapy and maintenance of range of motion. Early soft tissue coverage also decreases edema and pain.[8] Lister and Scheker[9] recommend immediate coverage, although this approach mandates aggressive debridement of all potentially nonviable tissue. Common indications for flap coverage of the elbow and forearm are listed in **Box 1**.

Box 1
Common indications for elbow and forearm soft tissue reconstruction

- Contracture release
- Trauma with exposure of bone, joint, tendon, or neurovascular structures
- Prosthetic exposure or prevention of prosthetic exposure
- Infection-related wounds
- Tumor extirpation-related wounds
- Autoimmune disease-related wounds

FASCIOCUTANEOUS FLAPS

The versatility and availability of axial fasciocutaneous flaps have made them a popular option for reconstructing wounds of the upper extremity. These flaps provide adequate soft tissue coverage, good contour, multiple possible orientations for flap inset, and a potential gliding surface for tendons.[10–13] In addition, fasciocutaneous flaps leave virtually no functional deficit[12,13] and secondary contouring is technically straightforward.[14]

Clinical Scenarios

Radial forearm pedicle flap
A 19-year-old right-hand–dominant man presented to the emergency department after falling 15 feet from a ladder, landing directly on his left elbow. Fractures of the left supracondylar humerus and distal radius were noted, as was the inability to extend the wrist and fingers. He underwent open reduction and internal fixation (ORIF) of the humerus and distal radius fractures, and a completely transected radial nerve was subsequently reconstructed with interposition nerve grafts. Provisional wrist extension was achieved with a simultaneous pronator teres to extensor carpi radialis brevis tendon transfer. Two months postoperatively, the humerus hardware became exposed, requiring washout, wound debridement, and hardware removal, resulting in a large, complex, elbow wound (**Fig. 2**A). The wound was successfully closed with a proximally based radial forearm flap (see **Fig. 2**B–D).

Discussion

The radial forearm flap was first described in 1978 by Yang and colleagues[15] and introduced to the West by Song and colleagues[16] as the "Chinese Flap" in 1982. This flap is considered one of the most reliable and versatile flaps for both pedicle and free flap reconstruction.[17] Owing to its long

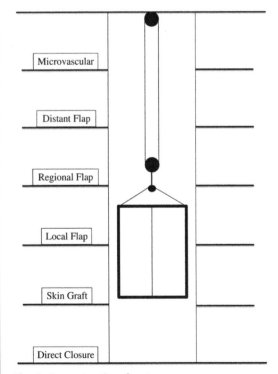

Fig. 1. Reconstructive elevator.

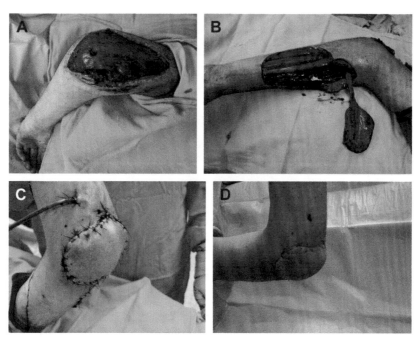

Fig. 2. Radial forearm pedicle flap. (*A*) Elbow wound after debridement. (*B*) Proximally based radial forearm flap. (*C*) Flap inset into wound. (*D*) Postoperative result.

pedicle, pliable soft tissue,[18] and ease of dissection, the radial forearm flap is a primary option in upper extremity reconstruction. The radial forearm can be harvested as either a fasciocutaneous or a fascia-only flap and can be used for small- and medium-sized defects of the dorsal elbow, the antecubital fossa, and in selected proximal forearm wounds. Alternative flaps should be strongly considered, however, in patients with traumatic injury to the volar forearm or an incomplete superficial palmar arch as noted by a preoperative Allen test.

The axis of the flap is from the central antecubital fossa to the radial styloid.[8] The proximally based flap used in elbow reconstruction relies on the distal cluster of clinically relevant perforators arising from the radial artery.[19] After skin paddle design, a paratenon-sparing dissection proceeds toward the interval between the flexor carpi radialis (FCR) and the brachioradialis tendons. Before distal radial artery ligation, it is prudent to confirm flow through the superficial palmar arch via the ulnar artery.[20] Donor-site closure frequently requires skin grafting, particularly if the flap is larger than 4 cm.[21] The muscle of the flexor digitorum superficialis can be used to cover exposed FCR tendon if paratenon is insufficient to support a skin graft.[1] Alternatively, a suprafascial dissection can be performed. This modification preserves the forearm fascia and

leaves a well-vascularized barrier of protection over the underlying tendons.[22]

In this case, a large and complex wound of the posterior elbow resulted from debridement and hardware removal. The radial forearm flap is an excellent option to close large wounds in this area. As a fasciocutaneous flap, it allows for early range of motion with thin, pliable coverage. It does, however, result in the division of a major artery to the hand and the comorbidity of a skin-grafted donor site. The reverse lateral arm flap may have been considered, although the posterior radial collateral artery was likely compromised by the humerus fracture and fixation. Furthermore, the extent of previous dissection and undermining likely resulted in compromise of the main pedicle, the radial recurrent artery. Free tissue transfer is a reasonable option, but regional fasciocutaneous flaps are preferred when they can provide an adequate closure while also avoiding the use of microsurgical techniques.

Reverse lateral arm pedicle flap
A 65-year-old right-hand–dominant woman presented to the clinic with a 6-month history of a draining bursa on the right posterior elbow (**Fig. 3**A). Her medical history was notable for rheumatoid arthritis treated with methotrexate and prednisone. A computed tomography scan of the elbow indicated no osteomyelitis. Despite

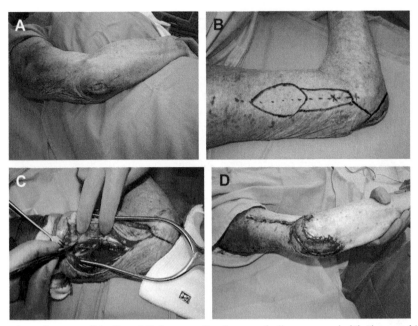

Fig. 3. Reverse lateral arm pedicle flap. (*A*) Preoperative image of elbow wound. (*B*) Flap markings. (*C*) Flap dissection. (*D*) Flap inset into wound.

treatment with antibiotics and hyperbaric oxygen, the wound did not improve. At an outside hospital, the wound was debrided and closed primarily. The patient noted wound separation with minimal trauma and requested a second opinion for wound closure. The wound was subsequently debrided and closed with a reverse lateral arm flap (see **Fig. 3**B–D).

Discussion

The lateral arm flap was described by Song and colleagues[23] in 1982. Although initially used as a free flap for head and neck reconstruction, the reverse pedicle modification has been successfully applied in soft tissue reconstruction of the elbow.[8] The lateral arm flap is supplied by the posterior radial collateral artery and has collateral flow through the radial recurrent artery in the proximal forearm.[24] The radial recurrent vessels provide inflow to the reverse lateral arm flap, with a lesser contribution from a recurrent branch of the posterior interosseous artery.[1] This flap may be contraindicated in the presence of trauma to the humerus or in obese patients.[25]

Flaps up to 8 × 15 cm have been described, although primary skin closure can be difficult if width exceeds 6 cm.[26] Elevation of the reverse lateral arm flap begins by marking the longitudinal axis between the deltoid and the lateral epicondyle.[27] Centering the flap on this line ensures that the vessels running in the lateral intermuscular

septum are captured during elevation. The flap is first dissected posteriorly, then anteriorly along the septum proceeding toward the humerus, with careful preservation of the radial nerve. Further dissection elevates the flap from the humerus in a proximal to distal direction after ligation of the proximal posterior radial collateral artery if used as a reverse pedicle flap for elbow coverage.

The reverse lateral arm flap is an excellent option for addressing small- to medium-sized posterior or lateral elbow wounds. It avoids the sacrifice of a major artery (see radial forearm flap) and provides adequate soft tissue for coverage of bone and neurovascular structures. Muscle flaps are not optimal in this location because they can adhere to underlying structures. Of the available options, the reverse lateral arm flap remains the simplest and also avoids the use of microsurgical free tissue transfer.

Free anterolateral thigh free flap

A 53-year-old left-hand–dominant man presented to the emergency department after sustaining a crush injury to his right forearm and wrist while clearing an auger used to dispense salt from a truck. Examination revealed an open dislocation of his distal radioulnar and radiocarpal joints, a distal radius fracture, and extensive soft tissue injuries to his forearm. He was taken to the operating room for initial debridement and external fixation of distal radioulnar and radiocarpal dislocations. After further debridement (**Fig. 4**A), ORIF of the

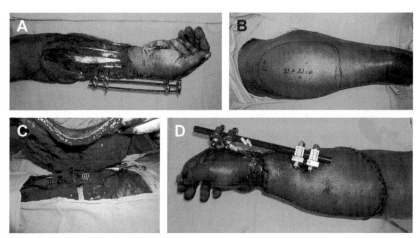

Fig. 4. Anterolateral thigh free flap. (*A*) Extensive forearm and hand wound after debridement. (*B*) Flap markings. (*C*) Flap elevation before transfer. (*D*) Flap inset into wound.

distal radius fracture and free anterolateral thigh (ALT) flap coverage of the forearm wound were performed (see **Fig. 4**B–D).

Discussion

Song and colleagues[28] first reported the ALT free flap in 1984. Since that time, it has seen broad application in extremity, trunk, abdomen, and head and neck reconstruction.[29] The ALT flap is most frequently supplied by musculocutaneous perforators (80%) arising from the lateral circumflex femoral artery.[30,31] Variable pedicle anatomy,[32] however, can make dissection difficult. Recent studies have shown that the anteromedial thigh flap may be a useful alternative in patients with inadequate ALT flap perforators discovered intraoperatively.[33]

Perforators typically arise within 3 cm of the midpoint between the anterior superior iliac spine and the lateral patella. If the perforator is septocutaneous, dissection proceeds quickly in the interval between the rectus femoris and vastus lateralus. The dissection necessarily proceeds more slowly if the perforator is musculocutaneous. In this frequent situation, meticulous technique is required to trace the pedicle through the vastus lateralus.[29,34] The donor site can generally be closed primarily.

Massive wounds of the forearm frequently require free tissue transfer, because no local options are available to provide appropriate coverage of exposed tendons and neurovascular structures. The ALT flap offers ideal characteristics to address the wound described in this case. Muscle or myocutaneous flaps (eg, latissimus dorsi flap) also would have achieved the goal of wound coverage. This option, however, would have compromised

motion and resulted in difficulty with flap elevation for secondary procedures. Pedicle 2-stage options (eg, thoracoabdominal flaps) for extensive forearm wounds result in a large donor site, often requiring skin graft closure, which can lead to a substantial aesthetic deformity and joint stiffness from prolonged immobilization.

MUSCLE AND MYOCUTANEOUS FLAPS

Muscle flaps can offer the advantage of dead space obliteration and significant soft tissue coverage with the ability to conform to irregular contours. Conflicting evidence exists regarding the advantage of muscle flaps compared with fasciocutaneous flaps in the setting of open fractures or contamination and osteomyelitis.[35,36] Experimental evidence suggests improved osseous healing and resistance to infection with muscle flaps,[35,37,38] although outcomes studies in humans show no statistical difference.[39,40] Furthermore, muscle flap elevation for secondary surgery can be difficult. When harvested as a pure muscle flap, a skin graft is mandatory and results in an additional donor site. Despite these disadvantages, multiple reliable muscle or myocutaneous flap options have been used successfully for both elbow and forearm wounds.

Clinical Scenarios

Flexor carpi ulnaris pedicle flap
A 26-year-old man was seen in the plastic surgery office for follow-up after sustaining 50% partial- and full-thickness burns to the torso and upper extremities in a house fire. On examination, a fixed left elbow flexion deformity was noted (**Fig. 5**A) associated with heterotopic ossification. The patient was taken to the operating room for excision

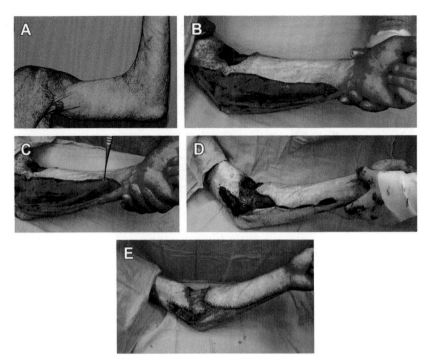

Fig. 5. Flexor carpi ulnaris pedicle flap. (*A*) Elbow flexion contracture. (*B*) Elbow and forearm wounds after burn contracture release. (*C*) Flexor carpi ulnaris muscle insertion divided and held in forceps. (*D*) Flexor carpi ulnaris muscle reflected proximally for medial epicondyle coverage. (*E*) Flap inset and skin graft placed.

of the burn scar, removal of heterotopic ossification at the medial epicondyle, ulnar nerve transposition, flexor carpi ulnaris (FCU) pedicle flap, and skin graft coverage (see **Fig. 5**B–E).

Discussion

The FCU muscle is located superficially in the forearm, making dissection straightforward. The dominant blood supply arises from the ulnar artery, with a smaller contribution from the posterior ulnar recurrent artery.[41] The FCU is innervated by the ulnar nerve and acts to flex and ulnarly deviate the wrist.[3] This flap is useful for small- to medium-sized defects of the elbow.

The axis of the flap is centered on a line from the medial epicondyle and the pisiform.[8] With a pivot point approximately 6 to 8 cm from the elbow flexion crease, the flap can be rapidly dissected after division at the musculotendinous junction.[1] The FCU can also be split into its 2 heads, retaining 1 for wrist flexion and ulnar deviation.[42] This technical modification may prove useful in patients anticipated to return to normal function after surgery.

In dealing with previously reconstructed burn wounds of the upper extremity, it is important to consider that local fasciocutaneous flaps (ie, radial forearm, reverse lateral arm) may have been compromised during tangential excision and skin graft closure. Both the FCU and brachioradialis muscle flaps will provide efficient coverage of small- to medium-sized wounds of the antecubital fossa or posterior elbow in this situation. A pedicle or free latissimus dorsi muscle flap would have provided more soft tissue than necessary to close the wound, while also requiring more difficult intraoperative patient positioning. Free fasciocutaneous flaps (eg, ALT) may be used for closure but require microsurgical expertise and equipment.

Brachioradialis pedicle flap

A 71-year-old right-hand–dominant man was referred to the plastic surgery clinic with a non-healing wound of the left posterior elbow (**Fig. 6**A). The elbow had been debrided 1 year before evaluation for an infected bursa requiring prolonged use of intravenous antibiotics. The wound had been managed with a vacuum-assisted closure in the interim. The patient was taken to the operating room for wound excision and a pedicle left brachioradialis muscle flap closure (see **Fig. 6**B, C). The skin was closed directly over the muscle with a stable long-term outcome (see **Fig. 6**D).

Discussion

The brachioradialis is another workhorse flap for small- to medium-sized soft tissue reconstruction

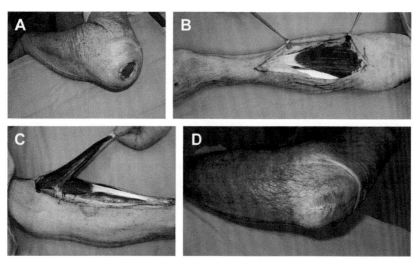

Fig. 6. Brachioradialis pedicle flap. (*A*) Preoperative image of elbow wound. (*B*) Flap dissection, sparing the dorsal radial sensory nerve. (*C*) Flap elevated. (*D*) Long-term result after primary closure over the flexor carpi ulnaris muscle flap.

at the elbow and can be elevated with minimal morbidity. It is the most superficial muscle on the radial aspect of the forearm originating proximally on the humerus between the brachialis and triceps.[3] At its origin, the brachioradialis is between 7 to 8 cm wide, and tapers distally providing approximately 15 cm of muscle.[43] The blood supply arises from the radial artery, the radial recurrent artery, or both.[44]

The muscle is exposed through a longitudinal incision over the proximal forearm. The musculotendinous junction is then divided and the muscle reflected proximally, revealing the pedicle approximately 10 cm distal to the origin. Extreme care is taken to preserve the dorsal sensory branch of the radial nerve.[7] Muscle transposition to the wound is technically easier if the origin is elevated off of the humerus.[1] The muscle flap can then be inset and covered with a split-thickness skin graft, if necessary.

Multiple local and regional options are available to address wounds in this location. Because no appreciable skin deficit resulted from wound excision, a regional muscle flap was sufficient to provide durable, well-vascularized soft tissue under the skin closure. The brachioradialis is an excellent option in this situation as a result of the minimal functional deficit incurred after elevation. The FCU muscle flap is an alternative option and a reverse lateral arm flap is useful when a skin deficit exists.

Latissimus dorsi free flap

A 32-year-old right-hand–dominant woman presented to the emergency department after a motor vehicle collision. On examination of the left upper extremity, the forearm skin was degloved from the elbow to distal forearm and the hand was well perfused. A distal radius fracture was noted on radiograph. The patient was taken to the operating room for debridement of the wound and external fixation of a comminuted and intra-articular distal radius fracture (**Fig. 7**A). At debridement, the FCU and flexor digitorum profundus tendons were discovered to be avulsed at their musculotendinous junctions. As such, the extensor carpi radialis longus tendon was transferred to the flexor digitorum profundus to maintain finger flexion. The wound was subsequently closed with a latissimus dorsi muscle free flap and split-thickness skin grafts (see **Fig. 7**B–D).

Discussion

The latissimus dorsi muscle originates from the lower 6 thoracic vertebrae, thoracolumbar fascia, and the iliac crest, converging to insert on the bicipital groove of the humerus.[45] The dominant vascular pedicle arises from the thoracodorsal artery with segmental perfusion from multiple lumbar perforators.[4] With dimensions averaging 25 × 35 cm,[46] this flap is a versatile, reliable, and technically straightforward option for pedicle coverage of the elbow and proximal forearm[47] or free flap coverage of massive forearm defects.[48] The flap may also be used as a functional muscle transfer to restore elbow flexion or extension.[49,50] An alternative flap should be chosen in paraplegic or crutch-dependent patients, because muscle harvest would lead to functional disability.[3]

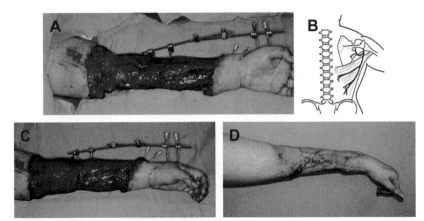

Fig. 7. Latissimus dorsi free flap. (*A*) Forearm wound after debridement. (*B*) Arterial anatomy of flap. (*C*) Free latissimus dorsi muscle flap after inset. (*D*) Long-term result.

With the patient in the lateral decubitus position, the incision is centered between the posterior axillary fold and the midpoint of the iliac crest. The skin flaps are raised, exposing the muscle that is then elevated off of the fascia and rhomboid muscles.[8] If used for pedicle soft tissue coverage, the insertion is left intact to prevent excess traction on the thoracodorsal artery during transposition and inset.[1] The donor site is closed primarily over a drain unless a skin paddle exceeding 10 cm has been harvested with the muscle, necessitating a skin graft for donor site closure.[45]

In this case, a massive forearm soft tissue defect was closed with a latissimus dorsi muscle free flap and skin graft. This flap is useful for muscle or myocutaneous coverage of large upper extremity defects, and effectively fills dead spaces. Although this achieved stable wound coverage, secondary contouring and tendon reconstruction is made simpler with fasciocutaneous flaps (eg, ALT). Despite this, the flap size requirement of a circumferential arm wound precludes the use of any standard fascial flap. Harvest of a flap with the dimensions necessary in this case would cause considerable donor site morbidity and also extend beyond the angiosome of the fascial flap pedicle. In situations requiring coverage of circumferential wounds with large dead spaces, flat muscle flaps, such as the latissimus dorsi or rectus abdominis, are good options. A thoracoabdominal pedicle flap may also be a reasonable option, but would result in a substantial donor site defect requiring a skin graft. This option also mandates multiple operations, while also leading to sequelae of immobilization.

DISTANT 2-STAGE PEDICLE FLAPS

Distant 2-stage pedicle flaps have a role when local and regional flaps are inappropriate or when recipient vessels for free tissue transfer are

in the zone of injury or absent.[51] Furthermore, distant pedicle flaps do not require microsurgical expertise and are a practical option when patient-related factors preclude the prolonged procedure times typical of microsurgical free tissue transfer.[3,52–55] These flaps can provide a large amount of skin and soft tissue for coverage of the forearm (up to 22 cm in length).[3] Distant flaps are used infrequently because of the immobilization required after flap inset, the need for several secondary operations, and prolonged length of hospitalization compared with free tissue transfer.[4,56]

Clinical Scenario

Intercostal artery perforator pedicle flap
A 7-year-old right-hand–dominant male presented with his parents to the hand surgery clinic 9 months after a right upper extremity crush injury sustained in an ATV accident. At the time of his injury, he underwent brachial artery reconstruction with a reversed saphenous vein graft at an outside hospital. His median nerve was transected but not reconstructed, and his wounds were closed with a combination of skin grafts and secondary intention. His parents desired evaluation of an elbow flexion contracture and an insensate thumb, index, and middle finger (**Fig. 8**A). He was taken to the operating room for excision of scar contracture and partial Z-plasty closure (see **Fig. 8**B), median nerve reconstruction with sural nerve grafts, biceps tendon lengthening, and intercostal artery perforator pedicle flap closure of the antecubital wound (see **Fig. 8**C, D). He returned to the operating room 4 weeks later for flap division, with a stable long-term outcome (see **Fig. 8**E).

Discussion

Pedicle thoracoabdominal flaps were first described in the 1940s.[57,58] The vast network of perforators

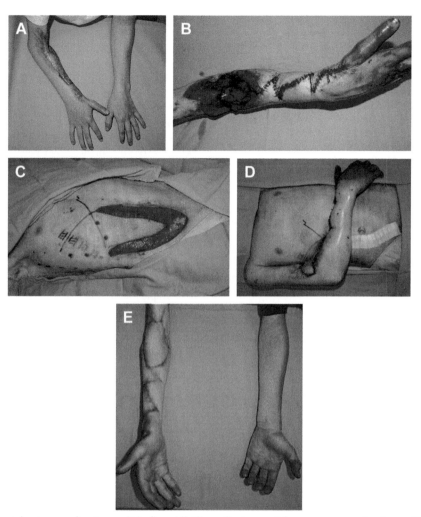

Fig. 8. Intercostal artery perforator pedicle flap. (*A*) Elbow flexion and forearm scar contractures. (*B*) Elbow and forearm wound after debridement and Z-plasty. (*C*) Flap design and elevation. (*D*) Flap inset. (*E*) Long-term result.

arising from the superior epigastric, inferior epigastric, deep circumflex iliac, intercostal, and subcostal arteries[59] provides a multitude of options for flap design and inset. Depending on size and orientation, thoracoabdominal flaps may have a random component,[60] particularly at the margins of larger flaps. These flaps are indicated in larger wounds of the forearm when microsurgical options are unavailable or contraindicated.

Free fasciocutaneous flap coverage of the wound seen in **Fig. 8**B would be an optimal choice. This technique was contraindicated in the setting of a previous brachial artery reconstruction. No local options were available that would offer sufficient and durable coverage over the exposed vital structures of the antecubital fossa. A latissimus dorsi muscle flap would have provided ample soft tissue. Secondary surgery would prove difficult after this flap, because

muscle flaps frequently adhere to underlying structures.

SUMMARY

Wounds about the elbow and forearm present unique anatomic and functional challenges for the reconstructive surgeon. The ultimate success of reconstruction relies on not only stable wound coverage but also early motion of adjacent muscles, tendons, and joints. Therefore, management requires a thorough understanding of the advantages and limitations of local, regional, distant, and free flap options. Patient-related and surgeon-dependent variables play an important role in determining the most appropriate flap choice for a given wound. Soft tissue coverage of the elbow and forearm can be successfully performed using the techniques presented.

REFERENCES

1. Giele H. Soft tissue coverage around the elbow. In: Stanley D, Trail I, editors. Operative elbow surgery: expert consult. London: Churchill Livingstone; 2012. p. 719.

2. Sharpe F, Stevanovic M, Itamura JM. Soft tissue coverage of the elbow. In: Mirzayan R, Itamura JM, editors. Shoulder and elbow trauma. New York: Thieme; 2004. p. 89.

3. Stevanovic M, Sharpe F. Soft-tissue coverage of the elbow. Plast Reconstr Surg 2013;132(3): 387e–402e.

4. Jensen M, Moran SL. Soft tissue coverage of the elbow: a reconstructive algorithm. Orthop Clin North Am 2008;39(2):251–64, vii.

5. Levin LS. The reconstructive ladder. An orthoplastic approach. Orthop Clin North Am 1993;24:393–409.

6. Bennett N, Choudhary S. Why climb a ladder when you can take the elevator? Plast Reconstr Surg 2000;105(6):2266.

7. Patel KM, Higgins JP. Posterior elbow wounds: soft tissue coverage options and techniques. Orthop Clin North Am 2013;44(3):409–17.

8. Moran SL, Johnson CH. Skin and soft tissue: pedicled flaps. In: Berger RA, Weiss AP, editors. Hand surgery. Philadelphia: Lippincott Williams & Wilkins; 2004. p. 1131–59.

9. Lister G, Scheker L. Emergency free flaps to the upper extremity. J Hand Surg Am 1988;13(1):22–8.

10. Pribaz JJ, Chan RK. Where do perforator flaps fit in our armamentarium? Clin Plast Surg 2010;37(4): 571–9.

11. Orgill DP, Pribaz JJ, Morris DJ. Local fasciocutaneous flaps for olecranon coverage. Ann Plast Surg 1994;32(1):27–31.

12. Fassio E, Laulan J, Aboumoussa J, et al. Serratus anterior free fascial flap for dorsal hand coverage. Ann Plast Surg 1999;43(1):77–82.

13. Geddes CR, Morris SF, Neligan PC. Perforator flaps: evolution, classification, and applications. Ann Plast Surg 2003;50(1):90–9.

14. Davami B, Porkhamene G. Versatility of local fasciocutaneous flaps for coverage of soft tissue defects in upper extremity. J Hand Microsurg 2011; 3(2):58–62.

15. Yang GF, Chen PJ, Gao YZ, et al. Forearm free skin flap transplantation. Chin Med J 1981;61:139–41.

16. Song R, Gao Y, Song Y, et al. The forearm flap. Clin Plast Surg 1982;9:21–6.

17. Lytle IF, Chung KC. Radial forearm flap. In: Rayan GM, Chung KC, editors. Flap reconstruction of the upper extremity: a master skills publication. Rosemont (IL): American Society for Surgery of the Hand; 2009. p. 97–105.

18. Jones NF, Jarrahy R, Kaufman MR. Pedicled and free radial forearm flaps for reconstruction of the elbow, wrist, and hand. Plast Reconstr Surg 2008; 121(3):887–98.

19. Saint-Cyr M, Mujadzic M, Wong C, et al. The radial artery pedicle perforator flap: vascular analysis and clinical implications. Plast Reconstr Surg 2010;125:1469–78.

20. Megerle K, Sauerbier M, Germann G. The evolution of the pedicled radial forearm flap. Hand (N Y) 2010;5(1):37–42.

21. Zenn MR, Jones GE. Reconstructive surgery: anatomy, technique, and clinical applications. St Louis (MO): Quality Medical Publishing, Inc; 2012. p. 855.

22. Lutz BS, Wei FC, Chang SC, et al. Donor site morbidity after suprafascial elevation of the radial forearm flap: a prospective study in 95 consecutive cases. Plast Reconstr Surg 1999;103(1):132–7.

23. Song R, Song Y, Yu Y, et al. The upper arm free flap. Clin Plast Surg 1982;9:27–35.

24. Prantl L, Schreml S, Schwarze H, et al. A safe and simple technique using the distal pedicled reversed upper arm flap to cover large elbow defects. J Plast Reconstr Aesthet Surg 2008;61(5): 546–51.

25. Sauerbier M, Geissler G. Lateral arm flap for hand wrist coverage. In: Moran SL, Cooney WP, editors. Soft tissue surgery: master techniques in orthopedic surgery. Philadelphia: Lippincott Williams and Wilkins; 2009. p. 179–80.

26. Slutsky DJ. Lateral arm flap. In: Rayan GM, Chung KC, editors. Flap reconstruction of the upper extremity: a master skills publication. Rosemont (IL): American Society for Surgery of the Hand; 2009. p. 189–94.

27. Tung TC, Wang KC, Fang CM, et al. Reverse pedicled lateral arm flap for reconstruction of posterior soft-tissue defects of the elbow. Ann Plast Surg 1997;38(6):635–41.

28. Song YG, Chen GZ, Song YL. The free thigh flap: a new free flap concept based on the septocutaneous artery. Br J Plast Surg 1984;37:149–59.

29. Wei FC, Jain V, Celik N, et al. Have we found an ideal soft-tissue flap? An experience with 672 anterolateral thigh flaps. Plast Reconstr Surg 2002; 109(7):2219–26.

30. Luo S, Raffoul W, Luo J, et al. Anterolateral thigh flap: a review of 168 cases. Microsurgery 1999; 19:232–8.

31. Kimata Y, Uchiyama K, Ebihara S, et al. Anatomic variations and technical problems of the anterolateral thigh flap: a report of 74 cases. Plast Reconstr Surg 1998;102(5):1517–23.

32. Lakhiani C, Lee MR, Saint-Cyr M. Vascular anatomy of the anterolateral thigh flap: a systematic review. Plast Reconstr Surg 2012;130(6):1254–68.

33. Yu P, Selber J, Liu J. Reciprocal dominance of the anterolateral and anteromedial thigh flap perforator anatomy. Ann Plast Surg 2013;70(6):714–6.

34. Wang HT, Fletcher JW, Erdmann D, et al. Use of the anterolateral thigh free flap for upper-extremity reconstruction. J Hand Surg Am 2005;30(4):859–64.

35. Chan JK, Harry L, Williams G, et al. Soft-tissue reconstruction of open fractures of the lower limb: muscle versus fasciocutaneous flaps. Plast Reconstr Surg 2012;130(2):284e–95e.

36. Tintle SM, Levin LS. The reconstructive microsurgery ladder in orthopaedics. Injury 2013;44(3): 376–85.

37. Gosain A, Chang N, Mathes S, et al. A study of the relationship between blood flow and bacterial inoculation in musculocutaneous and fasciocutaneous flaps. Plast Reconstr Surg 1990;86(6):1152–62.

38. Calderon W, Chang N, Mathes SJ. Comparison of the effect of bacterial inoculation in musculocutaneous and fasciocutaneous flaps. Plast Reconstr Surg 1986;77(5):785–94.

39. Hallock GG. Utility of both muscle and fascia flaps in severe lower extremity trauma. J Trauma 2000; 48(5):913–7.

40. Hallock GG. Relative donor-site morbidity of muscle and fascial flaps. Plast Reconstr Surg 1993; 92(1):70–6.

41. Payne DE, Kaufman AM, Wysocki RW, et al. Vascular perfusion of a flexor carpi ulnaris muscle turnover pedicle flap for posterior elbow soft tissue reconstruction: a cadaveric study. J Hand Surg Am 2011;36(2):246–51.

42. Wysocki RW, Gray RL, Fernandez JJ, et al. Posterior elbow coverage using whole and split flexor carpi ulnaris flaps: a cadaveric study. J Hand Surg Am 2008;33(10):1807–12.

43. McGeorge DD, Arnstein PM, Stilwell JH. The distally-based brachioradialis muscle flap. Br J Plast Surg 1991;44(1):30–2.

44. Leversedge FJ, Casey PJ, Payne SH, et al. Vascular anatomy of the brachioradialis rotational musculocutaneous flap. J Hand Surg Am 2001; 26(4):711–21.

45. Pierce TD, Tomaino MM. Use of the pedicled latissimus muscle flap for upper-extremity reconstruction. J Am Acad Orthop Surg 2000;8(5):324–31.

46. Chang LD, Goldberg NH, Chang B, et al. Elbow defect coverage with a one-staged, tunneled latissimus dorsi transposition flap. Ann Plast Surg 1994;32(5):496–502.

47. Vedder NB, Hanel DP. The mangled upper extremity. In: Green DP, Hotchkiss RN, Pederson WC, editors. Green's operative hand surgery. 6th edition. New York: Churchill Livingstone; 2011. p. 1634.

48. Bakri K, Moran SL. Initial assessment and management of complex forearm defects. Hand Clin 2007; 23(2):255–68, vii.

49. Stern PJ, Neale HW, Gregory RO, et al. Latissimus dorsi myocutaneous flap for elbow flexion. J Hand Surg Am 1982;7:25–30.

50. Hovnanian AP. Latissimus dorsi transplantation for loss of flexion or extension at the elbow. Ann Surg 1956;143:493.

51. Rockwell WB, Ley E. Abdominal flaps. In: Rayan GM, Chung KC, editors. Flap reconstruction of the upper extremity: a master skills publication. Rosemont (IL): American Society for Surgery of the Hand; 2009. p. 171–7.

52. Davis WM, McCraw JB, Carraway JH. Use of a direct, transverse, thoracoabdominal flap to close difficult wounds of the thorax and upper extremity. Plast Reconstr Surg 1977;60:526–33.

53. Fisher J. External oblique fasciocutaneous flap for elbow coverage. Plast Reconstr Surg 1985; 75:51–9.

54. Chow JA, Bilos ZJ, Hui P, et al. The groin flap in reparative surgery of the hand. Plast Reconstr Surg 1986;77(3):421–6.

55. Arner M, Möller K. Morbidity of the pedicled groin flap. A retrospective study of 44 cases. Scand J Plast Reconstr Surg Hand Surg 1994; 28(2):143–6.

56. Goertz O, Kapalschinski N, Daigeler A, et al. The effectiveness of pedicled groin flaps in the treatment of hand defects: results of 49 patients. J Hand Surg Am 2012;37(10):2088–94.

57. Brown JB, Cannon B, Graham WC, et al. Direct flap repair of defects of the arm and hand: preparation of gunshot wounds for repair of nerves, bones and tendons. Ann Surg 1945;122(4):706–15.

58. Cannon B, Trott AW. Expeditious use of direct flaps in extremity repairs. Plast Reconstr Surg 1949;4: 415–9.

59. Manahan M, Silverman RP. Chest and abdominal wall reconstruction. In: Guyuron B, Eriksson E, Persing J, editors. Plastic surgery: indications and practice. Philadelphia: Saunders Elsevier; 2009. p. 229–38.

60. Farber GL, Taylor KF, Smith AC. Pedicled thoracoabdominal flap coverage about the elbow in traumatic war injuries. Hand (N Y) 2010;5(1):43–8.

Free Muscle Flaps for Reconstruction of Upper Limb Defects

Mark V. Schaverien, MBChB, MRCS, MSc, MEd, MD, FRCSEng (Plast)[a],[*],
Andrew M. Hart, BSc, MBChB, MRCS, AFRCSEd, MD, PhD, FRCSEd (Plast)[b]

KEYWORDS

- Complex upper extremity injury • Timing of reconstruction • Free muscle flaps
- Functional muscle transfer • Reanimation • Indications

KEY POINTS

- Restoration of structure, function, and sensation after trauma or resection of tumor are critical in the hand.
- Early complete debridement, immediate repair/reconstruction of underlying structures and synchronous flap coverage enable early hand therapy, earlier return to function, and improved outcomes.
- In the upper limb, free tissue transfer is indicated for significant wounds around the elbow, forearm, and hand, where local options are inadequate, compromised by trauma, or would cause additional functional deficit or result in sacrifice of major axial vessels to the hand. Muscle flaps may also deliver functional reanimation.
- Muscle flaps contour well into complex three-dimensional defects, filling deep dead space. They may be indicated where the wound has been significantly contaminated or exposes a fracture (particularly with periosteal stripping/open joint).
- Commonly used free muscle flaps include the latissimus dorsi, rectus abdominis, gracilis, and serratus anterior flaps. The first 2 are commonly used as musculocutaneous flaps, and all may be split skin grafted.
- Postoperative rehabilitation is individualized for the structures injured. Active mobilization within 2 to 5 days of early debridement and reconstruction is desirable.

INTRODUCTION

Soft tissue defects are usually reconstructed by consideration of the reconstructive ladder, although the reconstructive elevator may be more appropriate for the upper limb to maintain dextrous, sensate interaction with surroundings. Superficial wounds can be managed by skin grafting, but in the hand, axilla, and antecubital fossa, there is a risk of secondary graft contracture, leading to restriction of movement and function, and aesthetic results may be unsatisfactory. Where underlying vital structures (eg, tendon, bone, nerve) are exposed, normal function requires

Funding sources: Mr M.V. Schaverien: none; Professor A.M. Hart: Stephen Forrest Charitable Trust.
Conflict of interest: none.
[a] Department of Plastic and Reconstructive Surgery, Ninewells Hospital, Dundee DD1 9SY, UK; [b] Canniesburn Plastic Surgery Unit, Glasgow Royal Infirmary, The University of Glasgow, Jubilee Building, 84 Castle Street, Glasgow G4 0SF, UK
* Corresponding author.
E-mail address: markschaverien@fastmail.fm

reconstruction with vascularized tissues. Flap cover enables early mobilization, which is critical to optimizing long-term function, and when local options are compromised (or would themselves compromise the outcome), early free tissue transfer from outside the zone of injury is required.[1–3] Thus complete debridement, repair, or reconstruction of vital structures, and primary free flap cover within approximately 24 hours of the injury is the ideal management for complex isolated upper extremity injury.[4]

Although primary amputation is frequently appropriate for severe lower limb trauma,[4,5] function with an upper limb prosthesis is generally poorer than after reconstruction, and upper limb amputation is associated with poorer health and psychosocial outcomes than limb salvage. Amputation may still be indicated after unrestorable devascularization injury, multicompartment muscle loss, if limb salvage would be life threatening,[6] or for the unreconstructable hand. A synchronous free flap may effectively preserve length on the amputation stump.[7] The optimal reconstruction is dependent on the mechanism and timing of injury, location and extent of wound contamination or infection, soft tissue and bone loss, the degree of nerve or tendon injury, the quality of vascular supply, and the suitability of the local tissues. When selecting a free flap, one must consider the flap dimensions, pedicle length/caliber, thickness, texture, color, durability, and sensory requirements. Donor site morbidity, facilitation of secondary reconstructive procedures, and surgeon's preference are also important.[1]

Early Complete Debridement

Tumor resection often requires composite tissue excision to obtain clear margins. A similar approach aids complex upper limb trauma management. For 12 to 24 hours after injury, wounds are typically necrotic and contaminated, rather than suppurative or subject to invasive infection. En bloc excision of this wound pseudotumor by sharp dissection through noncontaminated tissues and unbreached tissue planes is a critical part of flap reconstruction, by converting the contaminated wound into a fresh surgical wound, and is favored over serial debridement.[8–20] With the exception of critical, viable, longitudinal structures (nerves, vessels, tendons, viable bone), all dead, contaminated, or marginally viable tissue is removed, rendering the wound ready for immediate coverage (**Figs. 1–6**). Bacterial load is decreased, and a wound bed of healthy tissue facilitates flap survival, uncomplicated wound

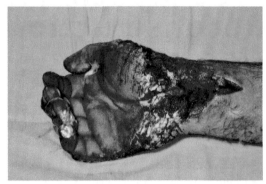

Fig. 1. Case 1: upper limb debridement series for a 38-year-old man involved in an industrial accident resulting in a crush/abrasion injury to the volar right wrist, radial and ulnar borders of the hand, and dorsum of the little finger. The patient presented 4 days after injury after exploration at a district general hospital. Debridement and reconstruction were undertaken with nerve graft reconstruction of the median nerve, and use of the palmaris longus tendon for reinsertion of abductor policis longus and extensor policis brevis tendons, as well as reconstruction of flexor carpi radialis tendon and the transverse carpal ligament. Synchronous free flap cover was used, using the radial artery and cephalic vein as recipient vessels. Palmar view of the preoperative wound, inadequately debrided, and with reactive extension of the zone of trauma and plaster of Paris contamination from inadequately applied dressings.

healing, and minimizes fibrosis. Furthermore, injured or missing structures can be clearly visualized and evaluated for primary repair or reconstruction.[18–20]

Reconstruction should be attempted as early as possible once adequate debridement is achieved. When adequate radical debridement is not possible, then, serial debridement is performed instead.[15]

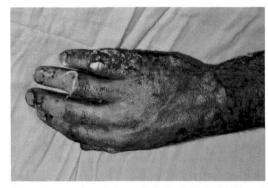

Fig. 2. Case 1: dorsal view of the preoperative wound, inadequately debrided, and with reactive extension of the zone of trauma.

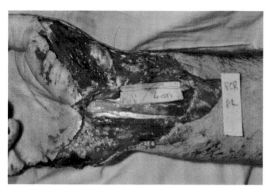

Fig. 3. Case 1: volar intraoperative view after adequate debridement showing a 4-cm segmental defect in the median nerve and palmaris longus tendon, a 3-cm defect in the flexor carpi radialis tendon, and intact radial and ulnar arteries.

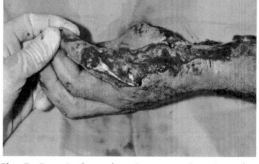

Fig. 5. Case 1: dorsoulnar intraoperative view after adequate debridement showing loss of most of the extensor mechanism to the little finger, and an open fifth metacarpophalangeal joint.

Immediate Flap Reconstruction

Three periods for reconstruction have been identified by Ninkovic and colleagues[21]:

1. Primary free flap cover is within 12 to 24 hours; longitudinal structures are repaired/reconstructed primarily, or bone injury is stabilized and reconstruction delayed.
2. Delayed primary free flap cover is between 2 and 7 days of injury; longitudinal structures are managed as above.
3. Secondary free flap cover is more than 7 days after injury, with delayed reconstruction of bone/longitudinal structures. Godina[9] first emphasized the advantages of early reconstruction, as well as the advantages of free flap over local flap techniques. Primary wound closure enables wound healing by primary

intention without the establishment of granulation tissue, fibrosis, and wound contracture. In the hand, it is also critical that mobilization is commenced at the earliest available opportunity to prevent joint stiffness, tendon adhesions, and soft tissue contracture compromising the long-term outcome.[19] Definitive reconstruction within the first 24 hours, when possible, was supported by Lister and Scheker[8] and by Chen and colleagues.[11]

Free tissue transfer provides the most appropriate repair for most severe injuries of the extremity; early transfer decreases infection risk, supports primary bone and soft tissue healing,

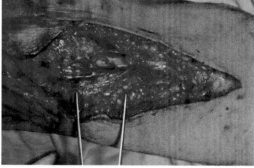

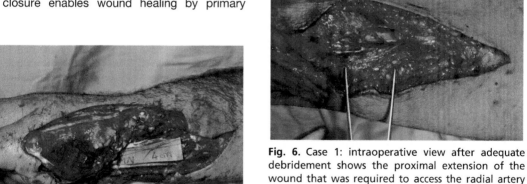

Fig. 4. Case 1: radial intraoperative view after adequate debridement showing an open carpometacarpal joint, exposed first metacarpal base denuded of periosteum, and segmental defects in the abductor policis longus (2 cm) and extensor policis brevis (3 cm) tendons.

Fig. 6. Case 1: intraoperative view after adequate debridement shows the proximal extension of the wound that was required to access the radial artery and cephalic veins outside the extended zone of trauma because of the delayed primary presentation. Note the change in the tissues from the edematous, bloodstained/hyperemic zone of trauma into the paler, healthy tissues. Decompression of the recipient vessels was then extended proximally in anticipation of the significant postoperative edema during the period of major fluid shifts that occurs during the postoperative care of free tissue transfers.

the commencement of early mobilization, and reduces inpatient hospital stay and overall costs.[7] Indications for immediate flap reconstruction are absolute and relative. Absolute indications include exposure of reconstructed or native major blood vessels and fillet-flap use of nonreplantable parts. Relative indications included the exposure of vital structures such as major nerves, joints, tendons without paratenon, and bone devoid of periosteum. Immediate reconstruction is contraindicated in unstable patients who cannot tolerate a prolonged operative procedure, in patients whose injuries are so severe that adequate debridement would destroy all possibility of meaningful function, in wounds with invasive infection, and in rare patients for whom amputation ± prosthesis would provide better function than reconstruction.[9,15–17]

Delayed Flap Reconstruction

Secondary free flap reconstruction delays rehabilitation, prolongs hospital stay, and increases overall costs and number of operations, although the initial operative time is shorter.[19,22] Granulation tissue develops in response to wound colonization, is poorly penetrated by antibiotics, and is a precursor to fibrosis.[23,24] Tissue edema peaks within 3 days of injury, and contributes to joint stiffness, fibrosis, inadequate mobilization, and extension of the physiologic zone of injury. Serial debridement may result in overall greater tissue loss caused by desiccation, extension of the zone of injury, and edema and granulation tissue compromising delineation between viable and nonviable tissue (see **Figs. 1–6**). The larger wounds that result from serial debridement, compared with primary debridement and reconstruction, make free tissue transfer more likely,[8] and longer pedicles necessary.[15]

A serial approach to debridement may be indicated in the unusual circumstance in which conversion of a contaminated wound to a cleaner wound is impossible, such as after severe crush injuries, severe multiplanar degloving, massive wound contamination, electrical burn injuries, or in patients with other life-threatening injuries that preclude a surgical procedure of required duration.

INITIAL REQUIREMENTS

On presentation with a severe upper limb injury, the patient should be managed according to advanced trauma life support principles, because there may be associated significant injuries. The neurovascular status of the limb should be carefully evaluated and documented before surgical intervention. The wound should be handled only for removal of gross contaminants, for photographic documentation, and to seal it from the environment. Radiographic assessment is performed, simple splintage applied, and antitetanus prophylaxis given if indicated. Broad-spectrum antibiotics (gram-positive and gram-negative cover) are administered in accordance with local policy as soon as possible, and continued at least until definitive soft tissue closure is obtained. Immediate surgical exploration may be indicated in the presence of gross contamination of the wound with agricultural, marine, or sewage contaminants, compartment syndrome, a devascularized limb, or in the multiply injured patient. In the operating room, the limb is washed with a soapy solution, and a tourniquet applied. The patient is positioned to facilitate flap harvest, and the limb prepared fully (an iodine solution stains tissue that needs to be excised). In the revascularized limb, blood supply may be temporarily restored by catheter first perfusion until soft tissue debridement and skeletal stabilization are performed.[25–27] Thorough wound debridement is performed under tourniquet control so that neurovascular structures can be clearly visualized and evaluated.[8,15–20] The tissues are systematically assessed by meticulous zone-by-zone debridement from superficial to deep (ie, skin, then fat, muscle, and bone), and from the periphery to the center of the wound, with all marginally and questionably viable tissue excised to convert a contaminated wound into a cleaner surgical wound.[8,14–20,28–31] Crushed and contaminated skin should be excised back to viable bleeding skin edges, and avulsed, contaminated, and devascularized subcutaneous tissue, fascia, and muscle should all be excised. Longitudinal structures in anatomic continuity, such as vessels with flow, nerves, and viable tendons are spared. Bone viability may be best assessed last, with tourniquet deflated. Small bony fragments providing no structural support are excised, whereas fragments with viable periosteum or attached articular cartilage are left in place. With the tourniquet deflated, any tissue that is not bleeding is re-excised until there is punctate bleeding with normal tissue encountered at all levels. Degloved tissue is carefully inspected and excised where clearly nonviable, but a second look within 24 hours may be required for nonviability to be declared before definitive reconstruction.

Wound lavage is performed with liberal amounts of Ringer lactate solution after debridement is completed, but high-pressure lavage is not recommended, because it may drive contaminants deeper into the wound and may damage vital structures.[32] If definitive soft tissue reconstruction is not performed at the time of debridement, then a topical negative pressure, or wet wound dressing, may be applied until reconstruction is performed. Antibiotic impregnated bone cement beads may be used where there is segmental bone loss.

After debridement, the wound is thoroughly examined to evaluate which anatomic parts are missing and what needs to be replaced. The objectives of reconstruction are not only to provide soft tissue coverage but most importantly to restore function. In deficits requiring coverage only, the size and depth of the wound are assessed, as well as the required vascular pedicle length. Where vital components are missing, the amount of missing bone, length of tendon defects, need for vein grafting, and the length of nerve gaps are also assessed. Primary reconstruction at the time of flap coverage is favored, although extensor tendon grafts should be deferred. The possibility of delivering primary reconstruction of functional elements from the flap, or its donor site, should be assessed (eg, flow-through or chimeric flaps). Any secondary reconstructions should be considered in relation to the choice of primary flap reconstruction.

Stable bony fixation is then applied where required and the wound then extended to allow access to recipient vessels outside the zone of injury where suitable local reconstructive options are not available. Deep veins are to be favored as recipients.

Principles of Debridement

- Best performed when necessary members of the care team are present, preferably within approximately 24 hours of injury
- Upper arm tourniquet control for bloodless field
- Sharp debridement through healthy tissue after tissue planes with sparing of longitudinal neurovascular structures
- Removal of foreign body contaminants
- Elimination of dead space by wider excision or transposition of local muscles without affecting function
- Bone debridement best performed with tourniquet deflated: small bone fragments with no structural support excised
- Completeness of debridement revaluated after tourniquet deflation, with punctate bleeding as end point, and further excision performed if necessary
- Copious low pressure irrigation with physiologic fluid (eg, Ringer lactate/normal saline)
- Samples taken for bacteriology before and after debridement

INDICATIONS

The patient should be stable and in a specialized center with appropriate microsurgical expertise. The wound should be adequately debrided and the limb well vascularized. Free flap reconstruction is indicated when suitable recipient vessels are present outside the zone of injury, where no suitable local pedicled flap option exists, where the defect is extensive,[8,9,15,28,33] or where a better overall functional and cosmetic outcome can safely be afforded. Free flaps should be favored over distant, staged, pedicled flaps, because completion in a single operative procedure enables the hand to be placed in the optimal resting position and mobilization to be commenced early, thereby minimizing fibrosis and stiffness. Free flaps are also nonsaprophytic, delivering well-vascularized tissue with angiogenic and lymphogenic potential to the wound.[2,34] Flaps may be part of a secondary reconstructive plan, or used for limb reanimation after muscle loss (usually proximal), or unrecovered motor nerve injury.

Soft tissue defects around the shoulder, axilla, and upper arm can often be reconstructed by pedicled muscle or skin flaps from the trunk. Smaller defects around the elbow and hand can be reconstructed using local skin flaps, but larger defects around the elbow, or in the forearm and hand, require free tissue transfer. Pedicled radial forearm flaps should be used with caution because the donor site is poor, an important vessel to the hand (and salvage free flap recipient vessel) is sacrificed, and significant aesthetic deformity may result.[7] Mutilating hand injuries are particularly amenable to free flap reconstruction because of the ability to transfer multicomponent vascularized tissues such as skin, fascia, bone, tendon, and nerve using chimeric flap techniques.

CHOICE OF FLAP

The fundamental requirement is that the selected flap has the necessary surface area and bulk to cover and obliterate the wound, pedicle length and caliber to match the recipient vessels, and is within the operating surgeon's competence. Knowledge of the mechanism of injury and degree of wound contamination allows the experienced operator to predict the size and depth of the wound after debridement (often significantly greater than the initial wound), which structures will be exposed (and require primary or secondary repair or reconstruction), and which recipient vessels will be available. The less experienced operator may need to complete the debridement and exploration of injured structures before finalizing the flap selection.

Flap selection should then be individually tailored to meet the operation logistics (eg, single/twin teams, positioning), to minimize the donor morbidity for that patient's specific requirements and optimize their cosmetic appearance and function (including sensory).[15,31,35–39] Planned secondary reconstructions should be facilitated and lifeboats not be burnt.

Options include skin flaps (perforator/fasciocutaneous flaps), musculocutaneous flaps or skin grafted muscle (±Integra [Integra LifeSciences Corporation, Plainsboro, NJ, USA][40]), or fascial flaps. In most cases, skin flaps are the most appropriate and may be available locally (movement around a perforator or pedicled). In the upper limb, it should be rare to require vein grafts (particularly in early debridement and reconstruction before reactive extension of the zone of trauma), within preference for flaps with inherently long pedicles (eg, anterolateral thigh flap can provide >12–15 cm pedicle as routine). Numerous recipient vessels are available in the upper limb, and several can be raised and transposed to obviate any need to use vein grafting.

In the upper limb, it is particularly important to ensure that the pedicle, anastomosis, and recipient vessels (particularly the veins) are not compressed, even if that necessitates dissection into the upper arm/axilla to release constricting overlying soft tissues and the use of skin grafts to cover the vessels at these points.

INDICATIONS FOR MUSCLE FLAPS, AND RATIONAL SELECTION

Cutaneous flaps provide the best sensory restitution (important in the hand), long-term pliability, tendon gliding, and appearance, and optimally facilitate secondary surgery.[39] Muscle flaps are pliable, can be trimmed, and separated or unfolded along their longitudinal fibers, and are therefore readily adapted into complex three-dimensional or deep wounds.[36–39,41] Although comparative clinical studies between muscle and perforator flaps after early debridement and modern fracture management are lacking for the upper limb compared with the lower limb,[42–46] muscle flaps may be favored for complex contaminated wounds and to fill in dead space.[21,29,47–51] Muscle flaps have been shown experimentally to have greater blood flow, antimicrobial activity, and biological contribution to bone healing than fasciocutaneous flaps.[52–56] Muscle flaps are necessary for reanimation (functional muscle transfer), a function that can be combined with wound coverage.

Although most upper limb muscles have been described as local flaps, most cover only a small area, and their harvest impairs limb function and should be avoided.[57] With the notable exception of the pedicled latissimus dorsi flap, which can resurface or reanimate large wounds to the level of the elbow, free tissue transfer is generally more appropriate if muscle flaps are to be used.

Musculocutaneous flaps deliver the benefits of both muscle and skin flaps if the circulation to the skin paddle is robust (eg, latissimus dorsi or rectus abdominis flaps), but can be bulky, in which case they should be harvested as muscle-only flaps and skin grafted. Integra may be applied directly onto the muscle and split skin grafted to provide a dermal layer and improve the cosmetic outcome.[40] Gliding tissues can be raised on separate pedicles (eg, latissimus dorsi flap (**Fig. 7**))[58] or released from the muscle surface after harvest (eg, gracilis flap). The distal perfusion in a musculocutaneous flap may be more reliable in the skin than the muscle, and the skin paddle can be raised and transposed based on a musculocutaneous perforator to increase coverage, decompress the pedicle, or during secondary operations.[1]

Muscle flaps are selected according to the size and depth of the defect, the required pedicle length/caliber, operative logistics, and individualized donor morbidity profile. Commonly used free muscle flaps include the latissimus dorsi, gracilis, rectus abdominis, and serratus anterior flaps, with the extensor digitorum brevis muscle used occasionally for small defects of the hand (**Table 1**).[59–64] The latissimus dorsi muscle is a workhorse flap for upper extremity reconstruction, because it provides a large surface area, reliable skin paddle, and long pedicle of good caliber (**Figs. 8** and **9**). Its harvest may require lateral decubitus positioning, cause persistent seroma unless the donor site is quilted, and compromise upper limb function for at least 6 weeks postoperatively.[65,66] The free flap should be preferentially harvested from the nondominant upper limb, and it should be used with caution in those with high functional demands of their upper limb. The rectus abdominis muscle also provides a large surface with a reliable skin paddle that can be designed with freedom of orientation and a long pedicle of large caliber; however, its harvest compromises abdominal wall function, although is generally well tolerated. The gracilis muscle flap is fast to raise, has an excellent donor site morbidity profile, and the epimysium can be incised to allow the muscle fibers to spread out and cover a relatively large surface area, but the pedicle is shorter. The serratus anterior muscle is recommended for

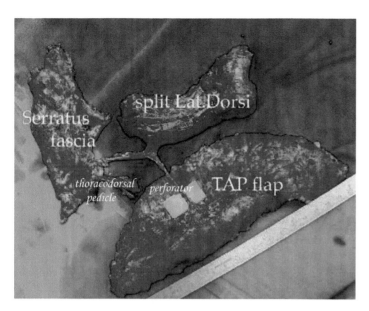

Fig. 7. Intraoperative view showing the chimeric flap principle based on the thoracodorsal pedicle. A compound flap is shown consisting of split latissimus dorsi muscle, a skin flap based on a thoracodorsal perforator, and a piece of serratus fascia, all joined together on the thoracodorsal pedicle. The serratus fascia can be used to provide a gliding plane over tendons, or to cover the flap pedicle. (*From* Van Landuyt K, Hamdi M, Blondeel P, et al. The compound thoracodorsal perforator flap in the treatment of combined soft-tissue defects of sole and dorsum of the foot. Br J Plast Surg 2005;58:374; with permission.)

digital reconstruction by some investigators (possessing multiple slips from 1 pedicle).

For functional muscle transfer, the pedicled latissimus dorsi and free gracilis flaps are well characterized for elbow reanimation (**Figs. 10–18**).[67] The gracilis muscle flap has been used to restore finger flexion/extension,[4] and for opposition (**Figs. 19 and 20**).[68]

Advantages of Muscle Flaps

- Straightforward anatomy, fast to raise
- Easy to inset into complex wounds
- Can provide large surface area coverage
- Obliterate deep wound dead space
- Better antimicrobial activity than fasciocutaneous flaps

- May improve fracture healing (particularly with periosteal stripping)

SURGICAL TECHNIQUE
Latissimus Dorsi Muscle Flap

Indications
The latissimus dorsi may be harvested as a muscle-only or musculocutaneous flap and is a workhorse pedicled flap for upper arm defects and free flap for defects of the forearm and hand. Based on the thoracodorsal artery via the subscapular artery, a pedicle length of up to 15 cm is achievable with an artery and single vein of 2 to 3 mm caliber (**Fig. 21**). The flap is relatively thin and pliable, and at ~20 × 40 cm in size reliably covers large defects (**Fig. 22**). Chimerism

Table 1
Summary of free muscle flap characteristics

Flap	Pedicle	Flap Size (cm)	Pedicle Length (cm)	Arterial Caliber (mm)
Latissimus dorsi	Thoracodorsal artery	20 × 40	Up to 15	2.0–3.0
Rectus abdominis	Deep inferior epigastric artery	10 × 30	5–7	2.0–4.0
Gracilis	Medial femoral circumflex artery	5 × 30	6–8	1.2–1.8
Serratus anterior	Branch of thoracodorsal artery	10 × 12	≤15	2.5–4.0
Extensor digitorum brevis	Branches of lateral tarsal artery and branch of the dorsalis pedis	5 × 5	A very long pedicle may be achieved by continuation to the anterior tibial artery	0.5–2.0

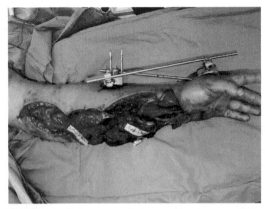

Fig. 8. Case 2: free extended musculocutaneous latissimus dorsi flap to cover a massive forearm wound from a high-energy crush injury in a 24-year-old man referred from an orthopedic center 2 days after debridement and external fixation of a compound fracture of the left radius and ulna. Preoperative volar view of the left forearm wound before examination under anesthesia, further debridement, and reconstruction with a free musculocutaneous latissimus dorsi flap. The use of tension sutures can be seen, which frequently serve only to further compromise tissue viability. Significant muscle necrosis was present in the long flexors, and a segmental median nerve defect was also present.

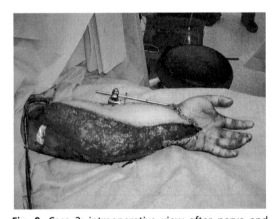

Fig. 9. Case 2: intraoperative view after nerve and muscle-tendon unit reconstruction, with synchronous cover with a free contralateral extended musculocutaneous latissimus dorsi flap, anastomosed end-to-side to the brachial artery, and end-to-end to a brachial vena comitans. The skin paddle was intentionally placed along the radial border of the wound to facilitate reelevation for planned secondary orthopedic surgery. The flap was raised in the deep subcutaneous facial plane to retain the deep fat over its surface, thereby optimizing the contour and reducing the likelihood of graft adhesion restricting the movement of underlying muscles. The remaining muscle flap was split skin grafted, with the expectation of serial excision in the future.

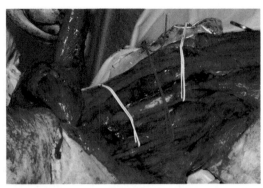

Fig. 10. Case 3: functional pedicled latissimus dorsi musculocutaneous flap reconstruction of the right arm in a 29-year-old right-hand-dominant man, employed as a roofer, who sustained a devascularizing compound fracture of the right humerus and clavicle as the result of a road traffic accident, with concomitant brachial plexus injury, in continuity injury of the radial, median, and ulnar nerves. Care before transfer included revascularization using saphenous vein graft reconstruction of the distal axillary artery, plate fixation of the humerus and clavicle, and preliminary debridement. Intraoperative view showing the vein graft reconstruction of the brachial artery (*middle sloop*), and the median and ulnar nerves (*left and right sloops*). The biceps muscle was confirmed to be nonviable and nonsalvageable, having been avulsed from its origins and from its vascular pedicle. A musculocutaneous latissimus dorsi flap was raised, having confirmed the intact subscapular axis. The flap was raised with a large skin paddle to restore the soft tissue defect, and with the gliding tissue layer between the latissimus and serratus anterior muscles raised on a branch of the thoracodorsal vessels.

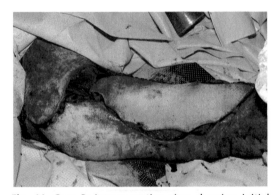

Fig. 11. Case 3: intraoperative view showing initial insetting of the flap. The tendon of the latissimus muscle was inserted onto the coracoid process, and the muscle was tubularized around the biceps tendon under tension, with the elbow flexed to 90°, with the forearm fully supinated. The chimeric element (gliding tissues) was used to wrap around the injured median and ulnar nerves, thereby isolating them from the damaged wound bed, preventing scar entrapment and facilitating gliding during rehabilitation.

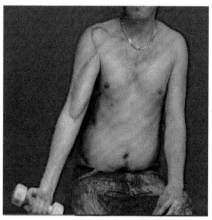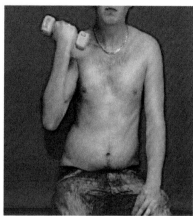

Fig. 12. Case 3: long-term outcome, by which time the patient had returned to work as a roofer, and could lift more than 5.5 kg weights in series of more than 10 repetitions.

with gliding tissues, the serratus anterior, scapular, or parascapular flaps permits reconstruction of more massive or complex wounds, and the use of vascularized bone (apex or lateral border of scapula, or rib segment) is possible (**Fig. 23**). The predictable branching of the thoracodorsal artery into descending and transverse branches allows splitting of the muscle in the line of its fibers for reconstruction of irregularly shaped defects. The anatomy of the thoracodorsal pedicle

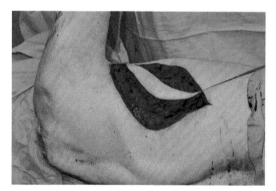

Fig. 13. Case 4: technique of functional pedicled latissimus dorsi musculocutaneous flap reanimation of elbow flexion in a 65-year-old patient presenting in her retirement with bilateral obstetric brachial plexus palsy, which included absent biceps function and elbow flexion in the right upper limb. Harvest of the musculocutaneous flap; the skin paddle is designed in reverse, and used for monitoring and to decompress the flap inset. The paddle should be placed over the thoracodorsal artery perforators toward the lateral border to the flap, not the distal/medial aspect. Dissection over the muscle is in the plane superficial to the muscle fibers to retain a thin gliding layer over the muscle to facilitate function. The lateral border is dissected first to confirm the pedicle anatomy.

also facilitates use as a flow-through flap for limb revascularization. The thoracodorsal nerve enables pedicled functional reconstruction of external rotation of the shoulder (eg, after obstetric brachial plexus injury), or of elbow flexion, where it can deliver sufficient power to lift more than 5.5 kg, and has endurance to complete multiple repetitions. Furthermore, the thoracodorsal nerve enables independent motor control such that the transferred latissimus dorsi muscle can be subconsciously activated to flex the elbow entirely independently of any shoulder adduction/internal rotation (see **Figs. 10–18**). As a free flap, the latissimus dorsi can deliver functional reanimation of the forearm when neurosynthesis is performed to a donor nerve distally in the upper limb.

The long-term donor site morbidity is low, with its deficit well-compensated for by the teres

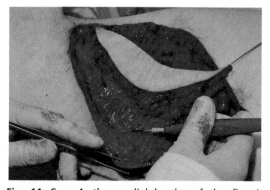

Fig. 14. Case 4: the medial border of the flap is released from the teres major, and the flap is released from the scapula. Care is taken to ligate the large lumbar and intercostal perforators at the underside of the flap.

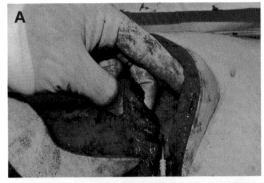

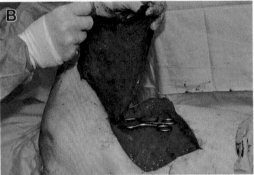

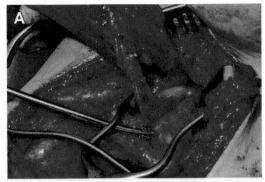

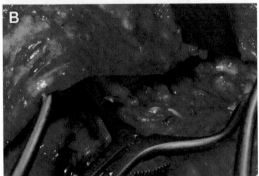

Fig. 15. Case 4. (*A*) The flap is then divided distally having taken care to ensure adequate length for biceps reconstruction, and (*B*) then the tendon is divided proximally under direct vision. For a functional latissimus flap, it is critical to raise the full length of the tendon, taking care to protect the nearby axillary vessels, brachial plexus, and radial nerve.

Fig. 16. Case 4: next, the thoracodorsal pedicle is dissected. In this case, the branch of the thoracodorsal pedicle (1 artery and 1 vena comitans) supplying the gliding tissues that separate the latissimus from serratus anterior has been ligated, as has the serratus branch to give greater reach (*A*). The thoracodorsal vessels and nerve are raised proximally, releasing bands of axillary fascia, until the circumflex scapular vessels are identified (1 artery, 2 venae comitantes) (*B*). For a free flap, dissection may not need to progress further, and the circumflex scapular artery can be preserved in many cases. For a pedicled flap to the arm, the circumflex scapular vessels should be divided to reduce the risk of pedicle kinking and venous occlusion.

major, although persistent seroma requiring aspiration is common unless quilting sutures are used, with or without the use of fibrin glue.[65,66] Quilting may be rapidly performed during donor site closure by placing interrupted 2/0 polydioxanone sutures (~10–15 in total) at intervals from the soft tissues of the chest wall into the Scarpa fascia of the donor site skin flaps (**Fig. 24**).

Anatomy

The flap originates from the posterior iliac crest, the thoracolumbar fascia, and the spinous processes of the lumbar and lower 6 thoracic

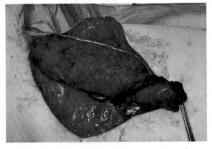

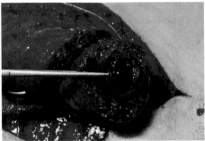

Fig. 17. Case 4. The flap has been tubularized to show the technique.

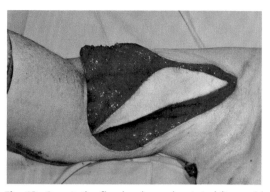

Fig. 18. Case 4: the flap has been derotated (to avoid pedicle torsion) and passed through a wide tunnel into the proximal arm. The tendon was inset onto the coracoid process using osseous sutures (or bone anchors). The distal flap was tubularized around the biceps tendon, with the elbow flexed to 90° and the forearm supinated. The skin paddle was then inset over suction drains and the arm splinted, with the elbow flexed, the forearm supinated, and the shoulder abducted to prevent venous compression. Tensioning of the flap affects the pedicle tension and risk of kinking/occlusion. Care should therefore be taken, and the pedicle checked before the final inset is completed.

vertebrae, and has a tendinous insertion into the intertubercular groove of the humerus. The subscapular artery arises from the axillary artery to run down the posterior axilla and split into the circumflex scapular and thoracodorsal vessels (see **Fig. 21**). The thoracodorsal vessels enter the undersurface of the flap within 5 to 8 cm of the musculotendinous junction with the

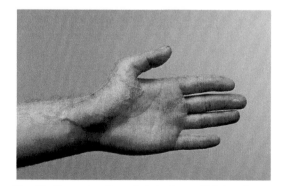

Fig. 19. Reconstruction of abductor pollicis brevis, opponens pollicis, and flexor pollicis brevis muscles of the left thenar eminence after crush-avulsion injury with a gracilis muscle flap and split skin graft and neural anastomosis to the recurrent motor branch of the median nerve. Note that there is restoration of the thenar bulk. (*From* Baker PA, Watson SB. Functional gracilis flap in thenar reconstruction. J Plast Reconstr Aesthet Surg 2007;60:831; with permission.)

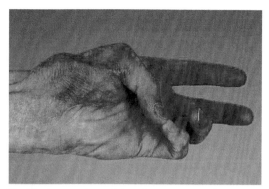

Fig. 20. Restoration of thumb opposition after gracilis muscle reconstruction of the thenar eminence. (*From* Baker PA, Watson SB. Functional gracilis flap in thenar reconstruction. J Plast Reconstr Aesthet Surg 2007;60:831; with permission.)

thoracodorsal nerve in close proximity, before splitting into descending and transverse branches.

Surgical procedure

The patient is placed in the lateral decubitus position, and the arm supported in well-padded supports to maintain ~90° of shoulder abduction and elbow flexion. The anterior border of the muscle and tip of the scapula are palpated and marked. Thoracodorsal artery perforators are marked using Doppler ultrasonography if a skin paddle is to be raised chimerically. Small lateral sections of the muscle can be raised supine.

An incision is made around the skin paddle (musculocutaneous flap; skin paddle is either aligned along the axis of the muscle or transversely) or border of the muscle (muscle-only flap), and the pedicle identified. Short-scar (6–10 cm) techniques are possible with the use of endoscopic or long instruments. Skin flaps are then raised off the muscle, the teres major separated away, its anterior margin raised, and the deep dissection completed. Care is taken not to raise the serratus anterior (laterally), paraspinal muscles (medially), or teres major (cranially), and to preserve the long thoracic nerve, before dividing the muscle medially and inferiorly (see **Figs. 13–15**). Under loupe magnification the vascular pedicle is isolated from the underside of the muscle and retrogradely dissected to the required pedicle length and caliber. The branch to serratus anterior and the circumflex scapular vessels may be divided to increase pedicle length (see **Fig. 16**). The muscle is divided proximal to the neurovascular hilum, or released from its tendinous humeral insertion (being aware of the neighboring radial nerve) for use as a functional transfer. When ready, the pedicle is divided, the

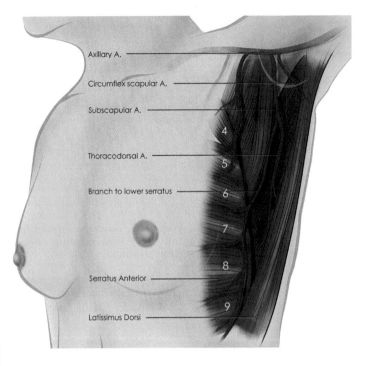

Axillary A.

Circumflex scapular A.

Subscapular A.

4

Thoracodorsal A.

5

Branch to lower serratus

6

7

8

Serratus Anterior

9

Latissimus Dorsi

Fig. 21. The anatomy of the subscapular arterial axis. The anatomic arrangement allows for chimerism with gliding tissues, the serratus anterior, scapular, or parascapular flaps, and vascularized bone from the apex or lateral border of scapula, or rib segment, enabling the reconstruction of large multicomponent defects, all based on the subscapular pedicle.

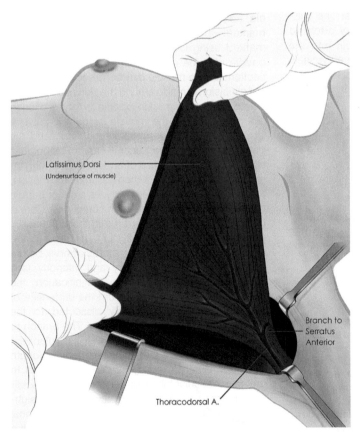

Latissimus Dorsi
(Undersurface of muscle)

Branch to Serratus Anterior

Thoracodorsal A.

Fig. 22. The harvest of a muscle-only latissimus dorsi flap via an incision at the anterior muscle border, showing the large surface are of flap that can be provided.

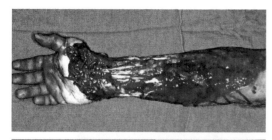

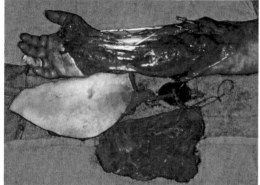

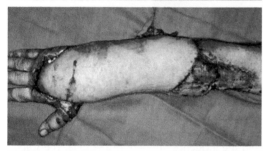

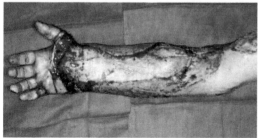

Fig. 23. Extensive circumferential degloving injury of the entire forearm resurfaced with a chimeric latissimus dorsi and scapular flap based on the subscapular system. (*From* Saint-Cyr M, Gupta A. Indications and selection of free flaps for soft tissue coverage of the upper extremity. Hand Clin 2007;23:46; with permission.)

donor site may be quilted, and then is closed in layers over 1 or 2 closed suction drains.

Rectus Abdominis Muscle Flap

Indications
The rectus abdominis muscle flap covers moderate-sized defects (**Fig. 25**). It may be harvested muscle only or with a transverse, vertical, or obliquely orientated skin paddle.

Anatomy
The paired rectus abdominis muscles, which are each up to 30 cm long and 10 cm wide, originate from the pubic symphysis and pubic crest to insert over the fifth to seventh costal cartilages. Above the arcuate line the muscle is enclosed by the rectus sheath, but it is found only anterior to the muscle below this. The deep inferior epigastric artery and vein originating from the external iliac vessels provide a reliable pedicle of more than 5 to 7 cm in length and 2 to 4 mm in caliber.

Surgical procedure
The muscle flap is most rapidly raised through a paramedian incision, deepened onto the rectus sheath, which is divided longitudinally and reflected using diathermy control of the musculocutaneous perforators (**Fig. 26**). The muscle is divided distally with ligation of the deep superior epigastric vessels, and proximally, at the required length, and the pedicle is dissected retrogradely from the lower lateral edge of the muscle until the desired length is achieved. The rectus sheath is then closed over an underlay prosthetic mesh or biological matrix using a continuous nonabsorbable suture and the wound closed in layers over a closed suction drain. The flap can be raised from a transverse incision along the pubic hairline using long instruments and lit retraction. The musculocutaneous flap should preferably be raised in a fascial sparing manner based on isolated perforators, to permit direct closure of the rectus sheath.

Gracilis Muscle Flap

Indications
The gracilis flap (muscle-only or musculocutaneous flap) is a workhorse for the coverage of small to medium-sized defects, with virtually no donor site morbidity; the skin paddle may be unreliable compared with other musculocutaneous flaps, which may be improved by raising a transverse skin paddle. When harvested with its motor branch of the obturator nerve for recipient-site neurosynthesis (up to ~15 cm is readily obtainable if the motor nerve is released from within the obturator nerve by intraneural dissection), the flap can also be used for functional reanimation of the elbow, wrist, or digits.

Anatomy
The gracilis is a long spindle-shaped muscle (~30 × 5–8 cm), which arises from the inferior pubic ramus, lies posteromedial to adductor longus, and inserts into the medial condyle of the tibia (pes

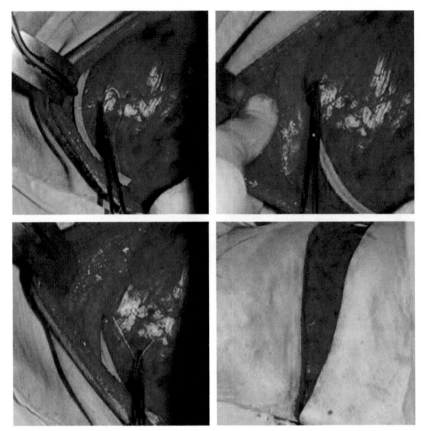

Fig. 24. Intraoperative series showing the process of quilting the latissimus dorsi muscle flap donor site. A series of interrupted 2/0 polydioxanone sutures are passed under vision from the soft tissue of the chest wall, into the Scarpa fascia of the donor site skin flaps, thereby immobilizing the skin over the chest wall to prevent shear and closing the dead space. This technique is effective at reducing the incidence of donor site seroma. The scapula should not be quilted to minimize the risk of shoulder dysfunction.

anserinus) (**Fig. 27**). The surface markings are generally more posterior than expected. The short (6–8 cm) pedicle arises from the medial circumflex femoral artery, with an arterial caliber of 1 to 2 mm and slightly larger paired venae comitantes, and enters the muscle at approximately 8 to 10 cm caudal to the pubic tubercle. A transverse or vertical skin paddle can be harvested of up to 20 × 10 cm, but requires care to ensure vascular reliability.

Surgical procedure

The patient is positioned supine, with the hip externally rotated and abducted, and knee flexed and supported. The thigh is prepared circumferentially to include the proximal third of the tibia, and the surface markings confirmed. A 10-cm longitudinal incision is extended from the adductor tubercle toward the medial femoral condyle, with a second incision made distally if the whole muscle length is required. The fascia over the adductor longus and gracilis is divided,

and the adductor longus retracted anteriorly to expose the neurovascular pedicle. Because the gracilis muscle lies more posterior than may be initially predicted, it is possible to erroneously raise the adductor longus. Early in the dissection, care should be taken to confirm the presence of longitudinal muscle fiber orientation and that the muscle extends/shortens during passive knee extension/flexion (when isolated from any hip movement). The surface of the muscle is dissected free, and the pedicle dissection commenced, taking care to avoid avulsion of a short branch to adductor longus, which is encountered early in the dissection. The deep surface of the pedicle, and the final 2 to 4 cm of its dissection, are best completed after dividing the muscle distally at the required length, after ligation of the minor pedicles from the femoral vessels; techniques for the blind division of the tendon insertion have been reported. The tendon of origin from the pubis is divided, and the wound is closed over a suction drain.

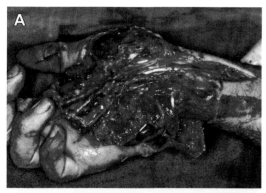

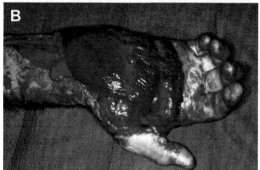

Fig. 25. Complex volar wrist and hand wound with exposure of flexor tendons and neurovascular bundles (*A*) resurfaced with a rectus abdominis muscle flap (*B*). (*From* Saint-Cyr M, Gupta A. Indications and selection of free flaps for soft tissue coverage of the upper extremity. Hand Clin 2007;23:47; with permission.)

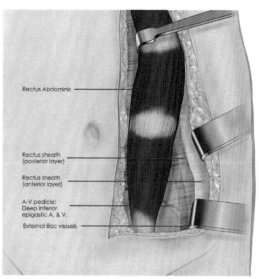

Fig. 26. Harvest of a rectus abdominis muscle flap. The muscle flap is most rapidly raised through a paramedian incision, deepened onto the rectus sheath, which is divided longitudinally and reflected using diathermy control of the musculocutaneous perforators. The muscle is then divided distally with ligation of the deep superior epigastric vessels, and proximally to the required length, with the pedicle dissected retrogradely from the lower lateral edge of the muscle until the desired length/caliber is achieved. The rectus sheath is then closed over an underlay prosthetic mesh or biological matrix using a continuous nonabsorbable suture, and the wound closed in layers over a closed suction drain.

Serratus Anterior Muscle Flap

Indications
The serratus muscle flap is based on the serratus branch of the thoracodorsal artery via the subscapular artery. The inferior 3 slips of the serratus muscle can be harvested to provide a thin flap that is suitable for resurfacing small and shallow defects. Donor morbidity is reportedly low, although the lower slips are prime scapular stabilizers during elevation of the arm. The flap may also be combined with a portion of vascularized rib or the latissimus dorsi muscle based on the common pedicle.

Anatomy
The serratus anterior muscle originates from the first 9 ribs and inserts onto the ventral surface of the medial border of the scapula. The lower 3 slips only are harvested, which have an independent blood supply from the serratus artery and neural supply from the long thoracic nerve (**Fig. 28**). A long pedicle length of up to 15 cm can be harvested if the subscapular artery is included, with an arterial diameter of up to 3 to 4 mm and a single vein.

Surgical procedure
With the patient positioned in the lateral decubitus position with the arm supported, an incision is made starting in the axilla over the anterior border of the latissimus dorsi muscle and curving anteriorly over the seventh to ninth ribs. This incision is continued through the subcutaneous fat to the latissimus dorsi muscle, which is then retracted laterally to expose the muscle origin and insertion. A plane is developed under the muscle and the attachments between the sixth and seventh slips divided, preserving the pedicle. The muscle slips are carefully dissected from the surfaces of the ribs, and the pedicle is then followed to the desired length before division of the insertion to the scapula. The donor site is closed in layers over a closed suction drain.

Other flaps that may occasionally be indicated include the extensor digitorum brevis muscle flap, the tensor fascia lata muscle flap, and the pectoralis minor muscle flap.

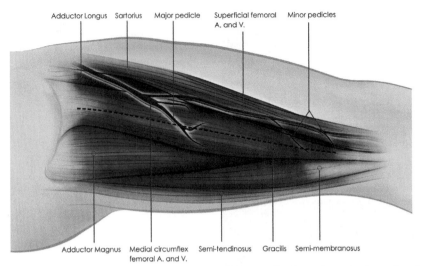

Fig. 27. The anatomy of the gracilis muscle. The gracilis is a long spindle-shaped muscle that arises from the inferior pubic ramus, lies posteromedial to adductor longus, and inserts into the medial condyle of the tibia as part of the pes anserinus. The surface markings are generally more posterior than expected. The short (6–8 cm) pedicle arises from the medial circumflex femoral artery and enters the muscle at approximately 8 to 10 cm caudal to the pubic tubercle. A transverse or vertical skin paddle can be harvested of up to 20 × 10 cm, but requires care to ensure vascular reliability.

PERIOPERATIVE CARE

Dressings should be bulky, with the first layers loosely applied to avoid external compression of the pedicle or anastomosis. Gauze dressings become more rigid or compressive with time (and egress of body fluids) and should be divided early if concern arises. One must also guard against kinking, first by avoiding the pedicle crossing joints where possible, and second, by

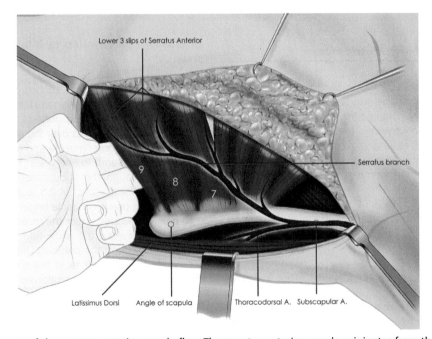

Fig. 28. Harvest of the serratus anterior muscle flap. The serratus anterior muscle originates from the first 9 ribs and inserts onto the ventral surface of the medial border of the scapula. The lower 3 slips only are harvested, which have an independent blood supply from the serratus artery and neural supply from the long thoracic nerve, and a long pedicle length of up to 15 cm can be harvested if continued to the subscapular artery.

careful splintage to control those joints during the early postoperative phase.

Splintage is applied to the theater dressing before recovering the patient according to the structures that have been repaired, and the course of the pedicle. Early mobilization (within 2–5 days, ideally) by hand therapists using a rehabilitation program individually tailored to the injury and specifics of the reconstruction optimize joint mobility, reduce swelling, and prevent tendon adhesions and soft tissue contractures.[3,39] Elevation on pillows is usually preferred to high elevation.

Primary free flap closure enables early introduction of a definitive rehabilitation program. Volar injuries involving flexor tendons are managed by early active mobilization protocols, and dorsal hand injuries involving extensor tendons are managed with static splintage for distal tendon injuries and with controlled active mobilization for proximal tendon injuries. As soon as wounds are suitable, a customized thermoplastic splint is fashioned, but straps must not compress the flap or its pedicle. Compression garments or bandaging should be introduced for muscle flaps once the skin grafts and wound healing are secure. Functional muscle transfers have a period of therapy to restore passive range, then others to learn muscle activation, to optimize force production and to dissociate motor control into normal cortical initiation pathways.

If delayed reconstruction is selected or necessary, then the optimal time for rehabilitation is lost, and the rehabilitation program is divided into 2 or 3 parts. Rehabilitation is first directed toward optimizing the passive range of movement, preventing tendon adhesions, controlling pain and swelling, and with splintage to prevent joint contractures. After secondary reconstruction, rehabilitation is continued to prepare the patient for definitive reconstruction. Final rehabilitation concentrates on functional recovery.

SUMMARY

Successful soft tissue reconstruction of the upper extremity with free flaps must be approached with the goals of not only providing stable coverage but most importantly of restoring function. The hand is poorly tolerant of prolonged immobilization, which predictably results in joint stiffness and tendon adhesions. Adequate debridement with immediate flap reconstruction at the earliest suitable opportunity and synchronous restoration of all missing tissue components (except extensor tendon grafts, which are best deferred) enable early mobilization and are the gold standard in suitable patients. Immediate wound closure, shorter hospitalization,

and avoidance of multiple procedures and multiple painful wound dressing changes are thereby facilitated.

Free flap reconstruction has many advantages in the upper limb, including versatility of flap design, reconstruction using well-vascularized tissue from outside the zone of injury, and avoidance of further morbidity to the injured limb. Although skin flaps are preferable for most applications, muscle flaps may conform better into large, or complex three-dimensional defects, are rapid, reliable, and straightforward to raise, and can reanimate lost motor functions. The latissimus dorsi and gracilis flaps can be adapted to meet most, if not all, requirements, and have good donor morbidity profiles.

Given the multitude of free flap options available to the reconstructive surgeon, flap selection should be based on the geometry of the defect, the required pedicle (to avoid vein grafting), patient factors, operation logistics, and intentions for reanimation or planned secondary surgery.

ACKNOWLEDGMENTS

The authors would like to thank Mark Roughley, Medical Artist at the University of Dundee, for providing the figures.

REFERENCES

1. Ninkovic M, Schoeller T, Wechselberger G, et al. Primary flap closure in complex limb injuries. J Reconstr Microsurg 1997;13:575–83.
2. Hing DN, Buncke HJ, Alpert BS, et al. Free flap coverage of the hand. Hand Clin 1985;1:741–58.
3. Saint-Cyr M, Gupta A. Indications and selection of free flaps for soft tissue coverage of the upper extremity. Hand Clin 2007;23:37–48.
4. Ninkovic M, Voigt S, Dornseifer U, et al. Microsurgical advances in extremity salvage. Clin Plast Surg 2012;39:491–505.
5. Higgins TF, Klatt JB, Beals TC. Lower Extremity Assessment Project (LEAP)–the best available evidence on limb-threatening lower extremity trauma. Orthop Clin North Am 2010;41:233–9.
6. Bray PW, Boyer MI, Bowen CV. Complex injuries of the forearm. Hand Clin 1997;13:263–78.
7. Hallock GG. The utility of both muscle and fascia flaps in severe upper extremity trauma. J Trauma 2002;53:61–5.
8. Lister G, Scheker L. Emergency free flaps to the upper extremity. J Hand Surg Am 1988;13:22–8.
9. Godina M. Early microsurgical reconstruction of complex trauma of the extremities. Plast Reconstr Surg 1986;78:285–92.

10. Godina M, Bajec J, Baraga A. Salvage of the mutilated upper extremity with temporary ectopic implantation of the undamaged part. Plast Reconstr Surg 1986;78:295–9.

11. Chen ST, Wei FC, Chen HC, et al. Emergency free-flap transfer for reconstruction of acute complex extremity wounds. Plast Reconstr Surg 1992;89:882–8.

12. Silverberg B, Banis JC Jr, Verdi GD, et al. Microvascular reconstruction after electrical and deep thermal injury. J Trauma 1986;26:128–34.

13. Chick LR, Lister GD, Sowder L. Early free-flap coverage of electrical and thermal burns. Plast Reconstr Surg 1991;89:10–9.

14. Breidenbach WC. Emergency free tissue transfer for reconstruction of acute upper extremity wounds. Clin Plast Surg 1989;16:505–13.

15. Gupta A, Shatford RA, Wolff TW, et al. Treatment of the severely injured upper extremity. Instr Course Lect 2000;49:377–96.

16. Scheker LR. Salvage of a mutilated hand. In: Cohen M, editor. Mastery of plastic and reconstructive surgery, vol. 3. Boston: Little, Brown; 1994. p. 1658–81.

17. Scheker LR. Soft-tissue defects in the upper limb. In: Soutar DS, editor. Microvascular surgery and free tissue transfer. London: Edward Arnold; 1993. p. 63–77.

18. Ninkovic M, Deetjen H, Ohler K, et al. Emergency free tissue transfer for severe upper extremity injuries. J Hand Surg Br 1995;20:53–8.

19. Sundine M, Shecker LR. A comparison of immediate and staged reconstruction of the dorsum of the hand. J Hand Surg Br 1996;21:216–21.

20. Scheker LR, Langley SJ, Martin DL, et al. Primary extensor tendon reconstruction in dorsal hand defects requiring free flaps. J Hand Surg Br 1993;18:568–75.

21. Ninkovic M, Mooney EK, Ninkovic M, et al. A new classification for the standardization of nomenclature in free flap wound closure. Plast Reconstr Surg 1999;103:903–14.

22. Scheker LR, Ahmed O. Radical debridement, free flap coverage, and immediate reconstruction of the upper extremity. Hand Clin 2007;23:23–36.

23. Burke JF. Effects of inflammation on wound repair. J Dent Res 1971;50(2):296–303.

24. Robson MC, Edstrom LE, Krizek TJ, et al. The efficacy of systemic antibiotics in the treatment of granulating wounds. J Surg Res 1974;16(4):299–306.

25. Pederson WC. Upper extremity microsurgery. Plast Reconstr Surg 2001;107:1524–36.

26. Cavadas PC, Landín L, Ibáñez J. Temporary catheter perfusion and artery-last sequence of repair in macroreplantations. J Plast Reconstr Aesthet Surg 2009;62:1321–5.

27. Chin KY, Hart AM. Temporary catheter first perfusion during hand replantation with prolonged warm ischaemia. J Plast Reconstr Aesthet Surg 2012;65:675–7.

28. Shen T, Sun Y, Cao D, et al. The use of free flaps in burn patients: experiences with 70 flaps in 65 patients. Plast Reconstr Surg 1988;81:352–7.

29. Ninkovic M, Schoeller T, Benedetto KP, et al. Emergency free flap cover in complex injuries of the lower extremity. Scand J Plast Reconstr Surg Hand Surg 1996;30:37–47.

30. Brenner P, Lassner F, Becker M, et al. Timing of free microsurgical tissue transfer for the acute phase of hand injuries. Scand J Plast Reconstr Surg Hand Surg 1997;31:165–70.

31. Giessler G, Erdmann D, Germann G. Soft tissue coverage in devastating hand injuries. Hand Clin 2003;19:63–71.

32. Hassinger SM, Harding G, Wongworawat MD. High-pressure pulsatile lavage propagates bacteria into soft tissue. Clin Orthop Relat Res 2005;439:27–31.

33. Saint-Cyr M, Langstein HN. Reconstruction of the hand and upper extremity after tumor resection. J Surg Oncol 2006;94:490–503.

34. Lutz BS, Klauke T, Dietrich FE. Late results after microvascular reconstruction of severe crush and avulsion injuries of the upper extremity. J Reconstr Microsurg 1997;13:423–9.

35. Neumeister M, Hegge T, Amalfi A, et al. The reconstruction of the mutilated hand. Semin Plast Surg 2010;24:77–102.

36. Hegge T, Neumeister MW. Mutilated hand injuries. Clin Plast Surg 2011;38:543–50.

37. Neumeister MW, Brown RE. Mutilating hand injuries: principles and management. Hand Clin 2003;19:1–15.

38. Seal A, Stevanovic M. Free functional muscle transfer for the upper extremity. Clin Plast Surg 2011;38:561–75.

39. Herter F, Ninkovic M, Ninkovic M. Rational flap selection and timing for coverage of complex upper extremity trauma. J Plast Reconstr Aesthet Surg 2007;60:760–8.

40. Moore C, Hart AM, Lee S, et al. Use of Integra for coverage of free muscle flaps. Br J Plast Surg 2003;56:66–9.

41. Wolff KD, Stiller D. Functional aspects of free muscle transplantation: atrophy, reinnervation, and metabolism. J Reconstr Microsurg 1992;8:137.

42. Heller L, Levin LS. Lower extremity microsurgical reconstruction. Plast Reconstr Surg 2001;108:1029–41.

43. Byrd HS, Cierny G 3rd, Tebbetts JB. The management of open tibial fractures with associated soft tissue loss: external pin fixation with early flap coverage. Plast Reconstr Surg 1981;68:73–82.

44. Pollak AN, McCarthy ML, Burgess AR. Short-term wound complications after application of flaps for coverage of traumatic soft-tissue defects about the tibia. The Lower Extremity Assessment Project (LEAP) study group. J Bone Joint Surg Am 2000; 82:1681–91.

45. Guzman-Stein G, Fix RJ, Vasconez LO. Muscle flap coverage for the lower extremity. Clin Plast Surg 1991;18:545–52.

46. Mathes SJ, Alpert BS, Chang N. Use of the muscle flap in chronic osteomyelitis: experimental and clinical correlation. Plast Reconstr Surg 1982;69:815–29.

47. Chang N, Mathes SJ. Comparison of the effect of bacterial inoculation in musculocutaneous and random-pattern flaps. Plast Reconstr Surg 1982; 70:1–8.

48. Najean D, Tropet Y, Brientini JM, et al. Emergency cover of open fractures of the leg. Apropos of a series of 24 clinical cases. Ann Chir Plast Esthet 1994;39:473–9.

49. Auclair E, Guelmi K, Selinger R, et al. Free transfer in the emergency treatment of complex injuries of the arm. Apropos of 18 cases. Ann Chir Plast Esthet 1994;39:338–45.

50. Foo IT, Malata CM, Kay SP. Free tissue transfers to the upper limb. J Hand Surg Br 1993;18:279–84.

51. Richards RR, Orsini EC, Mahoney JL, et al. The influence of muscle flap coverage on the repair of devascularized tibial cortex: an experimental investigation in the dog. Plast Reconstr Surg 1987;79:946.

52. Liu R, Schindeler A, Little DG. The potential role of muscle in bone repair. J Musculoskelet Neuronal Interact 2010;10:71–6.

53. Glass GE, Chan JK, Freidin A, et al. TNF-alpha promotes fracture repair by augmenting the recruitment and differentiation of muscle-derived stromal cells. Proc Natl Acad Sci U S A 2011;108: 1585–90.

54. Vogt PM, Boorboor P, Vaske B, et al. Significant angiogenic potential is present in the microenvironment of muscle flaps in humans. J Reconstr Microsurg 2005;21:517–23.

55. Gosain A, Chang N, Mathes S, et al. A study of the relationship between blood flow and bacterial inoculation in musculocutaneous and fasciocutaneous flaps. Plast Reconstr Surg 1990;86:1152–62.

56. Calderon W, Chang N, Mathes SJ. Comparison of the effect of bacterial inoculation in musculocutaneous and fasciocutaneous flaps. Plast Reconstr Surg 1986;77:785–94.

57. Him FP, Casanova R, Vasconez LO. Myocutaneous and fasciocutaneous flaps in the upper limb. Hand Clin 1985;1:759–68.

58. Takeishi M, Ishida K, Makino Y. The thoracodorsal vascular tree-based combined fascial flaps. Microsurgery 2009;29:95–100.

59. Del Piñal F, Pisani D, García-Bernal FJ, et al. Massive hand crush: the role of a free muscle flap to obliterate the dead space and to clear deep infection. J Hand Surg Br 2006;31:588–92.

60. Hatoko M, Muramatsu T. The use of latissimus dorsi muscle flap in the aesthetical reconstruction of heat-press injury of the hand. Burns 2001;27: 75–80.

61. Horch RE, Stark GB. The rectus abdominis free flap as an emergency procedure in extensive upper extremity soft tissue defects. Plast Reconstr Surg 1999;103:1421–7.

62. McGill D, Watson S. A novel use of the free gracilis muscle flap in hand trauma. Plast Reconstr Surg 2005;115:1801–2.

63. Topalan M, Ozden BC, Aydin A, et al. Use of free serratus anterior muscle slips for the reconstruction of dorsal-side defects of the hand resulting from hot press injury. J Burn Care Rehabil 2004;25: 346–8.

64. Del Piñal F, Herrero F. Extensor digitorum brevis free flap: anatomic study and further clinical applications. Plast Reconstr Surg 2000;105: 1347–56.

65. Sajid MS, Betal D, Akhter N, et al. Prevention of postoperative seroma-related morbidity by quilting of latissimus dorsi flap donor site: a systematic review. Clin Breast Cancer 2011;11:357–63.

66. Button J, Taghizadeh R, Weiler-Mithoff E, et al. Shoulder function after autologous latissimus dorsi breast reconstruction: a prospective two year observational study comparing quilting and non-quilting donor site techniques. J Plast Reconstr Aesthet Surg 2010;63:1505–12.

67. Kay SP, Pinder R, Wiper J, et al. Microvascular free functioning gracilis transfer with nerve transfer to establish elbow flexion. J Plast Reconstr Aesthet Surg 2010;63:1142–9.

68. Baker PA, Watson SB. Functional gracilis flap in thenar reconstruction. J Plast Reconstr Aesthet Surg 2007;60:828–34.

Indications, Selection, and Use of Distant Pedicled Flap for Upper Limb Reconstruction

S. Raja Sabapathy, MS, MCh, DNB, FRCS Ed, MAMS*,
Babu Bajantri, MS, MCh

KEYWORDS

- Pedicled flap • Soft tissue cover upper limb • Groin flap • Abdominal flap
- Hand injury reconstruction

KEY POINTS

- Pedicled flaps are easy to raise, are reliable, and do not need microsurgical expertise.
- Many of the disadvantages of pedicled flaps can be offset by properly planning the flap.
- Narrowing the base of the flap around the axial vessels, keeping just adequate length to allow comfortable mobility and primary thinning of the critical end of the flap are important steps.
- Good radical debridement before insetting of the flap facilitates primary reconstruction of tendons and bones.
- Secondary thinning can be aggressively performed in pedicled flaps.
- When vessels are not available for free flaps, or when free flaps fail, pedicled flaps can be a lifeboat.
- Pedicled flaps can also be used in preparation for a major microsurgical procedure, such as toe transfer or microsurgical bone reconstruction.

INTRODUCTION

The description of the pedicled groin flap by McGregor and Jackson[1] was a milestone in the journey of reconstruction of soft tissue defects of the hand. Understanding of the axial pattern of blood supply in that flap led to further identification of flaps based on various cutaneous vessels. Subsequent introduction of microsurgical free flaps enormously extended the reconstructive capability, to an extent that the option of a pedicled flap to cover soft tissue defects in the hand was often relegated to the background. Free flaps have the advantage of being a single-stage procedure, involve fewer hospital inpatient days, encourage the primary reconstruction of other injured structures, and patients do not have to go

through the discomfort and the period of "attachment" to the abdomen.[2]

Despite these advantages, pedicled flaps have survived as a valuable part of the reconstructive surgeon's armamentarium. Furthermore, refinements in techniques can offset most of the presumed disadvantages associated with pedicled flaps.[3] When well done, the outcome of pedicled flaps can be as good as and in certain aspects even better than what a free flap can achieve in the long term. In circumstances when free flaps cannot be done because of paucity of recipient vessels or infrastructural inadequacies or when they fail, pedicled flaps serve as lifeboats.[4]

In the reconstruction of complex defects, pedicled flaps can serve as a foundation for the subsequent microsurgical procedure. Groin flaps are

No disclosures for any of the authors.
Department of Plastic Surgery, Hand and Reconstructive Microsurgery and Burns, Ganga Hospital, 313, Mettupalayam Road, Coimbatore 641 043, India
* Corresponding author.
E-mail addresses: rajahand@vsnl.com; srs@gangahospital.com

Hand Clin 30 (2014) 185–199
http://dx.doi.org/10.1016/j.hcl.2014.01.002
0749-0712/14/$ – see front matter © 2014 Elsevier Inc. All rights reserved.

used to cover the amputation stumps of the fingers and thumb before toe transfers.[5] In major injuries and single vessel limbs, pedicled flaps are used to cover the soft tissue defect and subsequently the bone defect can be reconstructed with a free fibula transfer. In this way pedicled flaps are complementary to the success of microsurgery. Hence, it is mandatory on the part of an upper limb reconstructive surgeon to be well versed in the techniques of performing pedicled flaps. In most parts of the world they still serve as the workhorse in the management of upper limb injuries and will likely never be entirely supplanted by free tissue transfer.[6]

The anatomic basis of the commonly performed flaps, general principles that govern their use, site-specific technical considerations that influence the outcome, and complications and their avoidance are discussed in this article.

ANATOMIC CONSIDERATIONS

The infraumbilical part of the abdomen and the lateral aspect of the trunk serve as common donors of pedicled flaps. The lower part of the abdomen is supplied by three vessel branches that arise from the femoral artery and the paraumblical perforators (**Fig. 1**).

The superficial circumflex iliac artery (SCIA) arises from the femoral artery 2 cm below the

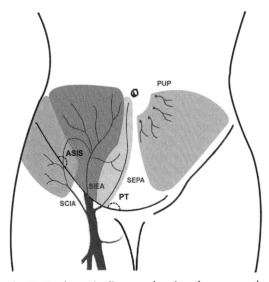

Fig. 1. A schematic diagram showing the commonly used flaps from the lower part of the abdomen for upper limb reconstruction and the vessels on which they are based. ASIS, anterior superior iliac spine; PUP, para umbilical perforators; SCIA, superficial circumflex iliac artery; SEPA, superficial external pudental artery; SIEA, superficial inferior epigastric artery.

inguinal ligament or from a common trunk along with the superficial inferior epigastric artery (SIEA). It then passes laterally and gives a deep branch at the medial border of Sartorius. The cutaneous branch becomes superficial at the lateral border of the Sartorius and runs into the tissue that is raised as the groin flap. The vessel runs parallel to the inguinal ligament, about 2 cm below it toward the anterior superior iliac spine. A simple "rule of two finger widths" has been recommended by Chuang and colleagues.[7]

The SIEA arises from the femoral artery 1 cm distal to the inguinal ligament and passes vertically upward superficial to the inguinal ligament within 2.5 cm of the midinguinal point. It soon becomes superficial by piercing the Scarpa fascia and runs superolaterally with the final branches traced up to the umbilicus.[8]

The superficial external pudental artery (SEPA) arises from the femoral artery close to the preceding branches and passes medially deep to the great saphenous vein toward the pubic tubercle.[9] It gives off branches at this point, and one of the branches ascends toward the umbilicus.

The deep inferior epigastric artery arises from the external iliac artery just proximal to the inguinal ligament, passes beneath the rectus abdominis muscle, and anastomoses with the superior epigastric artery within the rectus sheath. They give rise to perforators along their course that pierce the anterior rectus sheath to supply the skin. The highest concentration of these perforators is near the umbilicus and they feed into a subcutaneous vascular network that radiates like the spokes of a wheel.[10] These paraumbilical perforators are useful to raise flaps that are used for the reconstruction of the volar defects of the forearm.[11]

These are the main vessels on which pedicled flaps used for the upper limb are based. The branches of these vessels anastomose freely with each other in the anterior abdominal wall. Choke vessels exist between the territories and most often the dimensions exceeding the primary territory of a particular vessel can be raised by incorporating an adjacent territory. A flap of large dimension can be raised by incorporating these vessels in the base. The distance between the site of emergence of the SCIA and the SIEA into the subcutaneous tissue is only 6 to 8 cm in an adult, irrespective of the thickness of the abdominal wall (**Fig. 2**). By planning the base to include both the vessels, a flap of large dimensions involving the entire infraumbilical part of the lower abdominal wall up to the midline can be raised. This could also be raised as a bilobed flap to simultaneously cover the volar and the dorsal defects of the hand.[12,13]

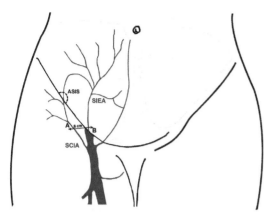

Fig. 2. Diagram illustrating the proximity of the sites of entry of the axial vessels of the groin flap and the hypogastric flap into the superficial plane. ASIS, anterior superior iliac spine. A, superficial external iliac artery; B, superficial inferior epigastric artery.

The lateral aspect of the chest and abdominal wall has a rich blood supply by perforators arising from the intercostal vessels and lumbar arteries. Flaps from the lateral part of the abdominal wall and trunk can be raised based on these vessels to cover the elbow and the proximal forearm.

GENERAL PRINCIPLES
Preparation of the Bed

Good debridement of the wound is the key to success. The basic plastic surgical principles, such as radical debridement and stable skeletal stabilization, must not be compromised. Attention to detail in the preparation of the bed must be the same whether one does a pedicled flap or an emergency free flap. Quality debridement should be performed even when a pedicled flap is planned. A flap on a good bed leads to a soft and supple flap, whereas a compromised bed leads to edema and induration of the flap.

Plan the Flap in Reverse

Comfort after inset of the flap is the main criteria for a successful outcome. The blood supply of the lower abdominal wall is good enough to allow one to plan the flap to cover any raw areas of the limb in a position of comfort. The hand or the part needing soft tissue cover is placed in a position of comfort and an appropriate flap of suitable dimensions is planned by making a pattern of the defect with a cloth piece or any pliable material. The flap can either be planned with the pedicle based superiorly or inferiorly as needed. For example, dorsal hand and forearm defects are easily covered by inferiorly based flaps based on

the superficial circumflex and SIEAs. Volar forearm defects are better managed by superiorly based flaps raised on the paraumbilical perforators. The technique of planning in reverse refers to marking the flap by following the steps in a reverse order (**Fig. 3**). "Measure twice, or thrice but cut once" is the key.

Keep the Base Narrow and Raise Custom Designed Flaps

The vessels on which these flaps are based are fairly constant in origin and course, so it is possible to keep the base narrow to include the vessels in the pedicle. By keeping the base narrow, the inset is increased and a flap to match the defect can be raised. If the base is broad, the flap does not match the defect and it results in bunching or unevenness of the flap at the time of suturing with cosmetically unacceptable results. Even large flaps can be raised by incorporating the SCIA, SIEA, and SEPA and the base could be as narrow as 8 cm (**Fig. 4**).

Keep Appropriate Length of the Pedicle

Adequate mobility depends on the length of the pedicle and is essential for comfort. Along with a small base, an adequate length of the pedicle allows movement of the flap-covered part during the postoperative period. It also facilitates therapy. Most of the time this idea is taken too far and a very long tubed pedicle is created. Too long a pedicle also results in the waste of well-vascularized tissue in the bridge segment and compromised blood supply in the distal end being attached to the defect. Most of the time we do not tube the pedicle; we just plan the pedicle length to allow supination and pronation of the forearm when the hand is being covered. There is a small raw area at the base of the pedicle that is dressed regularly. During division, the pedicle part of the flap is returned to cover the raw area and thus no valuable tissue is lost. Tubing the pedicle tightly can also cause edema of the flap.

Thin the Business End of the Flap

The SCIA, SIEA, and SEPA vessels course at a deep plane for a very short distance and they become progressively superficial and branch out into tissues that are raised as the flap. The distal part of the flap basically acts as a random pattern flap and survives exclusively on the subdermal plexus of vessels. Hence, this part of the flap could be radically thinned. This is the area that is inset into the defect and used for reconstruction and excellent aesthetic outcomes could be obtained by "relatively ruthless but careful" thinning of the

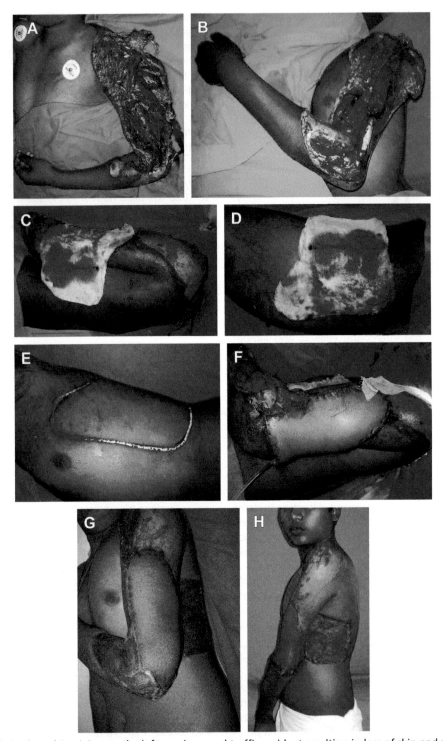

Fig. 3. (*A*) Crush avulsion injury to the left arm in a road traffic accident resulting in loss of skin and muscles on the lateral side with an open elbow joint and extensive contamination. (*B*) Postdebridement picture. (*C*) Planning in reverse: the arm is placed on the side of the body with the patient on the lateral side and a cloth piece marks the final flap required. (*D*) The arm removed and the pattern placed on the trunk and the flap marked. (*E*) The flap raised as per the mark and (*F*) inseted into the defect. The critical area is covered by the flap and the rest skin grafted. (*G, H*) Postoperative result. Patient had tendon transfers for the radial nerve loss and is back to all his activities.

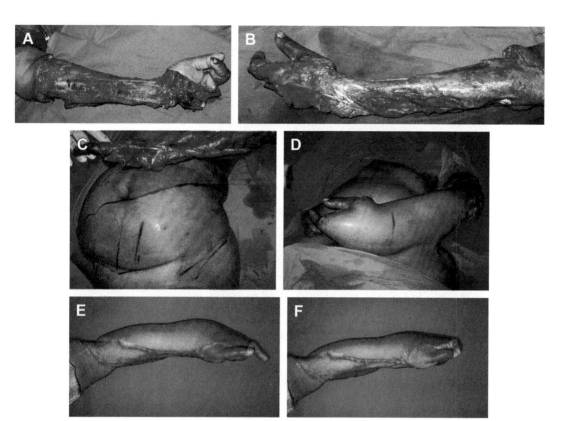

Fig. 4. (*A*, *B*) Major crush injury to the forearm and hand with circumferential skin and soft tissue loss with flap requirement along the whole length up to the metacarpal head. (*C*) Flap marked on the lower abdomen incorporating the groin flap, SIEA, and SEPA and opposite SEPA territory. (*D*) The flap raised keeping the SCIA, SIEA, and ipsilateral SEPA in the base. The small base helps to achieve good inset into the defect and the noncritical areas skin grafted. (*E*, *F*) Postoperative result with the thumb and the index finger fully functional.

flap.[14] This fact was emphasized very early on in the French literature by Colson and colleagues,[15] who raised skin flaps at the level of the subdermal plexus with virtually very little subcutaneous fat and found surprisingly large flaps can survive apparently entirely on this plexus. Even in obese individuals, the groin area is much thinner than the territories of the commonly used free flaps, such as the anterolateral thigh flap or the lateral arm flap. This fact combined with the techniques of primary thinning of the flap could result in a thin flap even in an obese individual.

Proximally the flap could be of full thickness in the pedicle part and the flap used to cover the defect can be thinned well. The flap is raised superficial to the external oblique aponeurosis initially and then thinned. This is because if the donor area needs to be covered with skin graft, the graft takes better on the fascia over the external oblique than on fat.

Bevel the Fat at the Skin Edge Before Inset

For ease of inset and better aesthetic appearance at the line of attachment, the fat at the skin edge is beveled (**Fig. 5**). A thick flap edge causes increased tension while suturing. Tight sutures cause unsightly suture marks and sometimes even necrosis of the edge of the flap.

Need for Delay Before Division of the Flap

During inset, if the flap is sutured to more than 80% of the perimeter of the defect, then the flap can be divided without a prior delay procedure before division. These flaps are well vascularized tissues and hence the flaps could be designed to fit the defect to increase vascular ingrowth. An aesthetically good outcome is thus obtained (**Fig. 6**). Often pedicled flaps get a bad reputation because of improper planning of the flap. It seems that the pedicle flap picks up more blood supply from the edges than from the base. This is probably because the fat on the underside of the flap is not a great interface to pick up blood supply from the bed. If the inset has less peripheral contact or the bed is infected then a prior delay is advised.

However, all tubed pedicled flaps must be delayed before division. Tubed flaps for osteoplastic

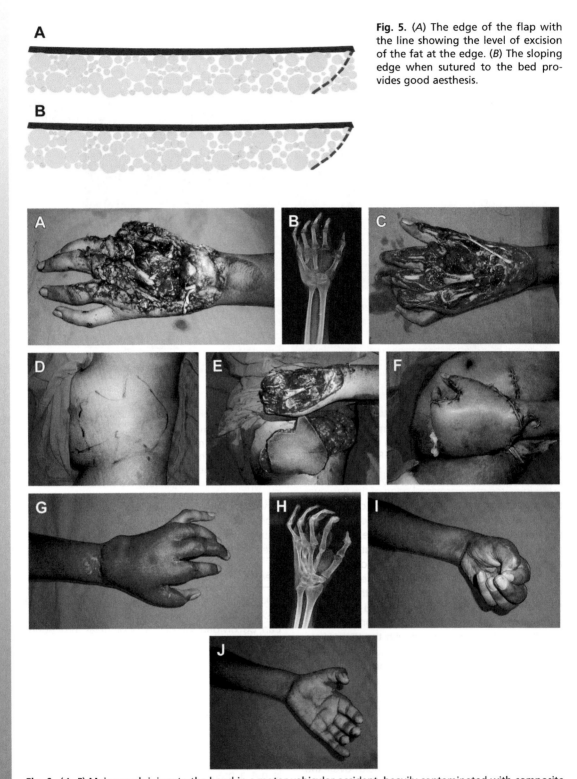

A

B

Fig. 5. (*A*) The edge of the flap with the line showing the level of excision of the fat at the edge. (*B*) The sloping edge when sutured to the bed provides good aesthesis.

Fig. 6. (*A, B*) Major crush injury to the hand in a motor vehicular accident, heavily contaminated with composite loss of skin, extensors, and the radiograph showing the bony loss. (*C*) The picture after debridement with the thumb positioned in an abducted and opposed position and the metacarpophalangeal joints in flexed position. (*D*) A custom designed flap marked incorporating both the groin and hypogastric flap vessels. (*E*) The flap raised. Note the small base of only 5 cm, which allows the flap to be rotated into the defect. (*F–J*) The final result with secondary iliac crest bone grafting and one round of thinning of the flap.

reconstruction of the thumb or to cover a circumferentially degloved finger must be delayed before division. The flap is divided 7 to 10 days after the delay procedure. Delay involves making an incision in the base of the flap and ligating or coagulating the main feeding vessels to the flap. Familiarity with the anatomy is helpful to identify the main vessel or Doppler can be used to find the location of the vessel.

Complex Primary Reconstruction with Pedicled Flaps for Cover

Emergency free flaps ushered in the era of complex primary reconstructions including primary bone and tendon grafting. There is always a lurking fear in the mind of the surgeon whether primary bone and tendon grafting is possible with pedicled flaps as cover. Early literature even recommended delayed cover of acute crushed hand injuries to decrease complications, such as infection, local tissue necrosis, and subsequent loss of flap.[16] With pedicled flaps, the pedicle proximal side is open and there is concern whether this could result in infection and failure. In our experience, this fear is unfounded (**Fig. 7**). We have treated 20 digits in 15 patients with dorsal combined tissue loss with radical debridement, primary nonvascularized iliac crest bone graft, and immediate abdominal flap cover. Eighteen of 20 digits achieved primary bone union and infection occurred in only one digit. Infection after bone grafting is related to the quality of debridement and stabilization of the fractures and early soft tissue cover.[17] It does not matter if the wound is covered by a free flap or a pedicled flap.

Anesthesia

We prefer the combination of brachial block and a subarachnoid block for the preparation of the hand and for the flap surgery. If the flap to be raised involves supraumbilical region the brachial block is combined with general anesthesia. Brachial block also helps in immediate postoperative pain relief.

SITE-SPECIFIC TECHNICAL CONSIDERATIONS
Flaps for the Fingers

There are few local flap options for cover for extensive raw areas in multiple adjacent fingers or circumferential raw area in a single finger. When it involves adjacent fingers, the fingers are temporarily syndactylized by covering with a pedicle flap. We usually prefer the hypogastric flap (based on SIEA) or the groin flap. The flap has to be custom designed and inset well into the proximal and distal ends of the raw areas. The pedicle has to be kept narrow to facilitate good inset. When the pedicle is well inset, flap division can be done at 3 weeks without delay and at the same time, syndactyl separation can also be done. Because of the fat content of the flap, the flap appears bulky on the dorsum of the fingers. The fat in the flap could be radically thinned at the time of syndactyly separation. Although it might look alarming, the flap usually survives with the distal and proximal skin attachment alone. Thus, it is important to obtain good approximation of the skin edges during the primary inset to make it possible. Thinning of the flap provides more skin to drape around the fingers. In case of residual raw areas in the margins, split skin graft is applied at the same sitting or a few days later when the thinned flap gets adherent to the bed (**Fig. 8**).

Sometimes a single finger may need a distant pedicle flap. This usually happens when there is composite tissue loss that requires primary reconstruction or would need secondary reconstruction. When a single finger is covered, the part is kept in the most comfortable position and flap raised. If we are including the named arteries in the base, then the base could be made narrow and the inset increased.

Tubed flaps are provided for cover of degloved fingers or as the first step for osteoplastic thumb reconstruction. The inset has to be adjusted in such a way that the flap points in the right direction. The flap draped around the finger must be thinned to make it aesthetically acceptable. All tubed flaps to a single finger must be delayed before division, because the skin attachment is proportionately less compared with the extent of the flap. Without delay there is unacceptable incidence of tip necrosis of the flap.

Flaps to the Hand

Both groin (SCIA based) and hypogastric (SIEA based) flaps could be used for the purpose. Our first preference is for the hypogastric flap because it is easy to raise and the base could be reliably made narrow. For dorsal defects it insets better. If the lower abdomen is fat, we prefer the groin flap. The same flap could be used to cover either the dorsum or the volar side by the way the donor area is narrowed or closed.[18] We use a key stitch in the base to turn the direction of the flap (**Fig. 9**). The donor area could be primarily closed if the width of the flap is less than 6 to 9 cm depending on the profile of the patient.

It is essential to plan and thin the flap so that appropriate contour is obtained. The inset can almost reach 90% for these flaps. If secondary

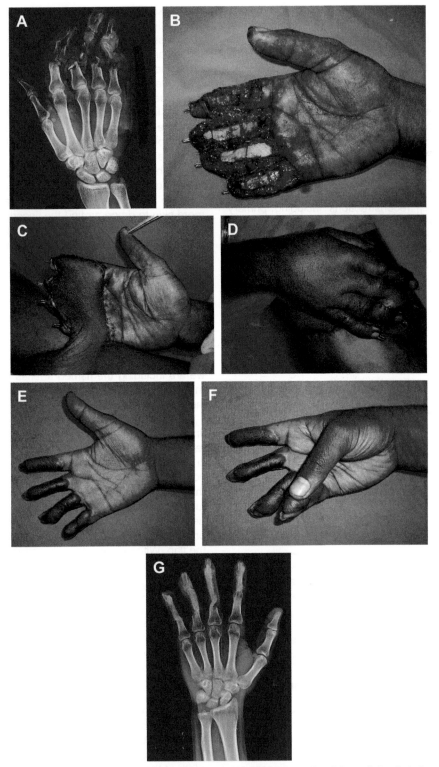

Fig. 7. (*A*) Radiograph of a textile machinery injury showing extensive loss of middle and distal phalanges. (*B*) The injury also resulted in loss of volar skin, flexors with viable dorsal skin up to the tip of the fingers. Fingers reconstructed with primary bone graft from the iliac crest and the fingers syndactalyzed before flap cover. (*C*) Flap designed to match the defect raised based on the SIEA and the donor area primarily closed. (*D*) Dorsal view. (*E–G*) Long-term pictures showing good outcome with good incorporation of the bone graft.

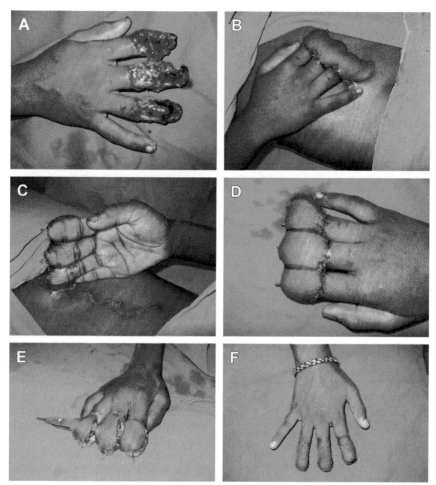

Fig. 8. (*A*) Dorsal composite loss in the distal segment of adjacent fingers. (*B, C*) Covered by hypogastric flap after syndactylization of the fingers with primary closure of the donor area. (*D*) The flap divided at 3 weeks without delay and immediate separation of syndactyly along the marked lines. (*E*) The flap thinned to the layer of the dermis with attachments only on the proximal and distal sides. (*F*) Long-term result.

tendon reconstruction is needed the flap is kept a little bulky for the passage of the tendon grafts through the fat. However, the flaps to the palm must be made as thin as possible so that grip is possible. A bulky flap in the palm is aesthetically unacceptable and functionally disabling. It acts as if the patient has already something in the hand.

When both the volar and dorsal defects have to be covered, a bilobed flap is planned. The groin and the hypogastric flap are raised in a bilobed manner on a single pedicle and each turned over to cover the hand, which is sandwiched between the two flaps. In such situations the groin flap covers the dorsum, whereas the hypogastric flap covers the volar defect (**Fig. 10**). This design can be combined with forearm flaps to primarily cover total degloving injuries of the hand.[19]

Flaps to the Forearm and for Combined Defects

When the soft tissue defect of the hand extends to the fingers or proximally into the forearm, large flaps can be raised by incorporating adjacent territories of the vessels. When all four vessels are included in the base, a large flap of 30 by 15 cm can be raised reliably without delay and it is enough to cover a defect extending from the elbow to the metacarpophalangeal joint of the fingers. The lateral margin goes up to the posterior axillary line and medially it can cross the midline up to the lateral margin of the rectus sheath of the opposite side. These flaps could be raised primarily without delay, but it is safer to delay such large flaps before division. Delay is done by dividing one-third of the flap on either side and the whole flap is divided and inset a week later.

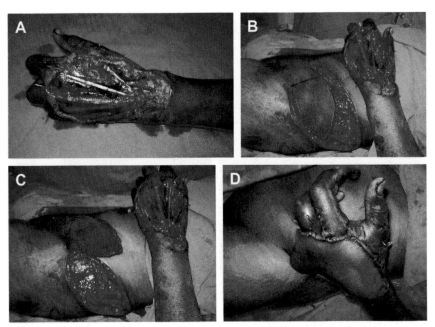

Fig. 9. (*A*) Defect on the dorsum of the hand. (*B*) Groin flap raised. (*C*) The closure technique resulting in the flap pointing to cover the defect. (*D*) The flap inset into position.

Flaps to the volar side of the forearm require meticulous planning. The flap is based on the paraumbilical perforators (**Fig. 11**).[20]

Flaps to the Elbow

This is a challenge for a reconstructive surgeon, particularly when it happens as part of a major high-velocity trauma, such as sideswipe injuries with associated comminuted fractures. Skeletal stability is of paramount importance before providing pedicled flap cover. The fixation quality has to be of a higher order than a free flap for cover. Loose skeletal fixation causes severe pain in the postoperative period. Internal fixation is our choice for all upper limb skeletal injuries and in the region of the elbow if there is some instability because of the comminution of the fractures or bone loss, an auxiliary external fixator is applied on the lateral side.

Flap planning is made easier by putting the patient on the lateral side. The arm and elbow are kept on the body in a comfortable position and the flap planned. For defects on the anterior side the flap is based anteriorly (**Fig. 12**) and for posterior defects a posteriorly based flap is designed. The perforators from the intercostal arteries and lumbar arteries are present along the midaxillary line and that is kept as the base of the flap. Donor area is skin grafted. When done in that position, we have found that the patient is very comfortable while walking and being in bed. On rare occasions

when the elbow needs circumferential cover, and if free flaps cannot be done, pedicle flaps can be planned. We have devised a technique for such instances whereby an anteriorly based trunk flap is used to cover the anterior defect. The donor area exposes the latissimus dorsi muscle and an inferiorly based latissimus dorsi muscle flap is raised to cover the posterior aspect of the elbow. The elbow is sandwiched between the skin flap anteriorly and muscle flap posteriorly. Trunk flaps are an easy and reliable technique for defects of the elbow extending from the distal third of the arm to the proximal third of the forearm. Yunchuan and colleagues[21] used lateral intercostal perforator-based pedicled abdominal flap for upper limb wounds from severe electrical injuries.

Defects proximal to the distal third of the arm are easily and better covered with pedicled latissimus dorsi or pectoralis muscle flaps.

Flaps in Children

Contrary to popular thinking, children do very well with pedicled flaps.[22] We have done pedicled abdominal flaps in children as young 4 months without any problem. One needs to restrain them when they come out of anesthesia, but once awake, they do exceptionally well. Children do not pull away the flaps because it causes pain. Nevertheless, the hand is restrained by elastocrepe bandage or tapes until the flap is divided. In our experience the children are discharged from

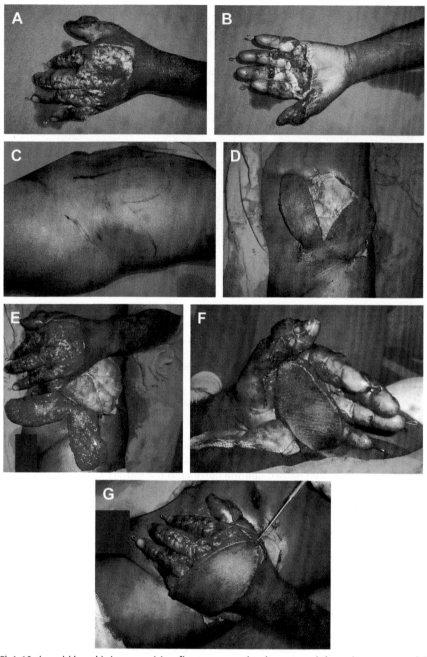

Fig. 10. (*A, B*) A 10-day-old hand injury requiring flap cover on the dorsum and the palmar aspect of the hand. (*C*) A bilobed flap marked, one a groin flap and the other the hypogastric flap on a common pedicle. (*D, E*) The raised flap, the donor area skin grafted, and the hand in preparation of inset. (*F*) The hypogastric flap used to cover the palm. (*G*) The groin flap covers the dorsum of the hand.

the hospital in 4 to 5 days and do very well at home (**Fig. 13**).

POSTOPERATIVE CARE

At the end of the procedure, the limb is immobilized by broad plaster tapes that restrain the patient from pulling the flap away from the body. It should also prevent kinking of the flap. This needs to be done irrespective of whether the procedure has been done under regional anesthesia or general anesthesia. Postoperative monitoring and adjustment are made easy by a technique that we follow.[23] After the correct position of

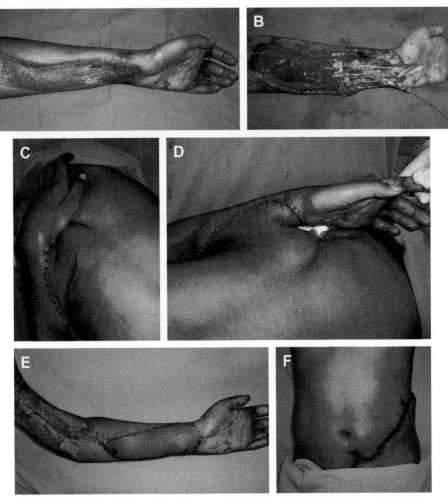

Fig. 11. (*A*) A patient with electrical burns sequelae with skin-grafted lower forearm needing flap cover for future reconstruction. (*B*) Skin graft excised and the nerve ends marked. (*C, D*) A superiorly based flap based on the paraumbilical perforators raised and inset into the defect. (*E*) Long-term result. (*F*) The donor area.

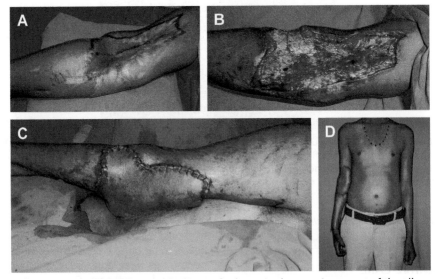

Fig. 12. (*A*) A patient with electrical burns with skin-grafted area in the anterior aspect of the elbow with loss of elbow flexors. (*B*) The skin graft excised. (*C*) An anteriorly based trunk flap has been given with the patient in the lateral position. (*D*) The long-term outcome. The patient subsequently had pectoralis major transfer.

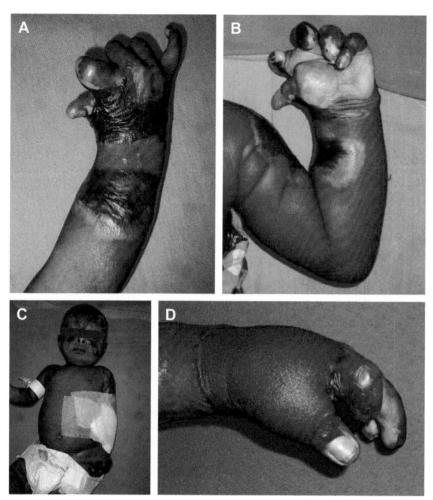

Fig. 13. (*A, B*) Severe postburn contracture of the hand in an infant. (*C*) The baby comfortable with the flap. The picture shows the type of restraint applied to the child in the immediate postoperative period. (*D*) The result showing the thumb functioning again.

immobilization is safeguarded by plaster restraints, three lines are drawn on the forearm and continued on to the abdomen. The patient and the relatives are instructed to keep the lines in continuity and that makes the whole process easier (**Fig. 14**). We remove the restraints after about 5 days, and we have not had any complications. In addition, the physiotherapist massages and mobilizes the shoulder and elbow and the wrist as much as possible. It is also possible to mobilize the fingers with the flap in situ in the immediate postoperative period. Patients usually are mobilized from the bed in 24 to 48 hours and are discharged when they are comfortable.

SECONDARY PROCEDURES
Thinning of the Flap

Pedicled flaps have the advantage over free flaps in that during secondary thinning, the entire flap can be thinned almost to the subdermal level. This is achieved by making small access incisions on the border of the flap at intervals and using the access to excise all the fat that is accessible to the

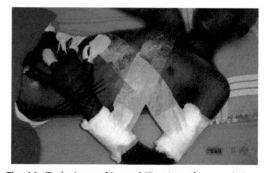

Fig. 14. Technique of immobilization after an abdominal flap. Note the three lines that run along the forearm and then on the abdomen of the patient to guide the patient and the family as to the hand position.

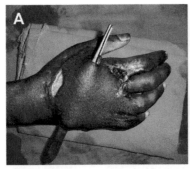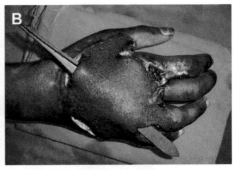

Fig. 15. (*A, B*) Technique of thinning of the flap. Small access incisions made to gain access and the whole flap can be thinned to subdermal level in a single sitting.

incision. By strategically placing the incisions the entire flap can be thinned in one sitting (**Fig. 15**). It is our estimate that up to one-third of the perimeter could be incised for access incisions and we have not had any problem.

Secondary Reconstructions Under the Flap

Edema in the flap and induration at the suture line settle in about 6 to 8 weeks after the flap inset. When the flap becomes supple and the induration at the suture line is reduced, the patient is ready for the secondary procedure. This is a better yardstick than to have a rigid time frame for secondary reconstruction. The flap is opened on one side for bone grafting. If tendon grafts are done it is better to tunnel them through the flap. The flap margins are the sites of maximum resistance for the passage of tendon grafts and also the site where tendon adhesions often occur. If we are aware of the need for secondary tendon reconstruction, great effort is taken to massage the scar line from the very beginning. We also provide custom-made compression garments to reduce the edema.

COMPLICATIONS

Necrosis of the flap is the worst complication one can have, but fortunately loss of the whole pedicle flap is very rare. Marginal necrosis can occur. The patient is conservatively treated if excision of the compromised flap would not expose a vital structure or another flap is considered.

Physiotherapy instituted immediately after the patient comes out of anesthesia helps to prevent stiffness of the joints. A good amount of patient counseling before the operation and spending some time with the patient in the immediate postoperative period encourages the patient to follow the therapy instructions. We divide the flap under brachial block and after division the shoulder is put through the whole range of movement. This mobilization under anesthesia is helpful to get them moving quickly.

SUMMARY

Pedicled flaps remain a valuable technique of soft tissue cover in upper limb reconstructive surgery. They are versatile, have less demand on infrastructure, and if technical refinements are practiced they also prove to be cost effective. Demands on the period of training, attention to detail, and skill in execution are no less than what a free microsurgical flap would need for success. Proficiency in pedicled flaps provides the hand surgeon a higher level of confidence when faced with a complex defect or when a free flap seems difficult or risky to execute.

REFERENCES

1. McGregor IA, Jackson IT. The groin flap. Br J Plast Surg 1972;25:3–16.
2. Goertz O, Kapalschinski N, Daigeler A, et al. The effectiveness of pedicled groin flaps in the treatment of hand defects: results of 49 patients. J Hand Surg Am 2012;37:2088–94.
3. Sabapathy SR. Refinements of pedicle flaps for soft tissue cover in the upper limb. In: Venkataswami R, editor. Surgery of the injured hand. New Delhi (India): JaypeePublishers; 2009. p. 131–8.
4. Mih AD. Pedicle flaps for coverage of the wrist and hand. Hand Clin 1997;13:217–29.
5. Sabapathy SR, Venkatramani H, Bhardwaj P. Reconstruction of the thumb amputation at the carpometacarpal joint level by groin flap and second toe transfer. Injury 2013;44:370–5.
6. Friedrich JB, Katolik LI, Vedder NB. Soft tissue reconstruction of the hand. J Hand Surg Am 2009; 34:1148–55.
7. Chuang DC, Colony LH, Chen HC, et al. Groin flap design and versatility. Plast Reconstr Surg 1989; 84:100–7.

8. Reardon CM, O'Ceallaigh S, O'Sullivan ST. An anatomical study of the superficial inferior epigastric vessels in humans. Br J Plast Surg 2004;57:515–9.

9. Patil UA, Dias AD, Thatte RL. The anatomical basis of the SEPA flap. Br J Plast Surg 1987;40:342–7.

10. Boyd JB, Taylor GI, Corlett R. The vascular territories of the superior epigastric and the deep inferior epigastric systems. Plast Reconstr Surg 1984;73:1–16.

11. Yilmaz S, Saydam M, Seven E, et al. Paraumbilical perforator based pedicled abdominal flap for extensive soft-tissue deficiencies of the forearm and hand. Ann Plast Surg 2005;4:365–8.

12. Smith PJ. The Y-shaped hypogastric-groin flap. Hand 1982;14:263–70.

13. Choi JY, Chung KC. Combined use of a pedicled superficial inferior epigastric artery flap and a groin flap for reconstruction of a dorsal and volar hand blast injury. Hand 2008;3:375–80.

14. McGregor IA. Flap reconstruction in hand surgery: the evolution of presently used methods. J Hand Surg 1979;4:1–10.

15. Colson P, Houot R, Gongolphe M, et al. Use of thinned flaps (flap grafts) in reparative hand surgery. Ann Chir Plast 1967;12:298–310.

16. Chow JA, Bilos ZJ, Hui P, et al. The groin flap in reparative surgery of the hand. Plast Reconstr Surg 1986;77:421–6.

17. Sabapathy SR, Venkatramani H, Giesen T, et al. Primary bone grafting with pedicled flap cover for dorsal combined injuries of the digits. J Hand Surg Eur 2008;33:65–70.

18. Bajantri B, Latheef L, Sabapathy SR. Tips to orient pedicled groin flap for hand defects. Tech Hand Up Extrem Surg 2013;17:68–71.

19. Doctor AM, Mathew J, Ellur S, et al. Three flap cover for total hand degloving. J Plast Reconstr Aesthet Surg 2010;63:e402–5.

20. O'Shaughnessey KD, Rawlani V, Hijjawi JB, et al. Oblique pedicled paraumbilical perforator based flap for reconstruction of complex proximal and mid-forearm defects: a report of two cases. J Hand Surg Am 2010; 35:1105–10.

21. Yunchuan P, Jiaqin X, Sihuan C, et al. Use of the lateral intercostal perforator-based pedicled abdominal flap for upper limb wounds from severe abdominal injury. Ann Plast Surg 2006;56:116–21.

22. Mathew P, Venkatramani H, Sabapathy SR. Mini-abdominal flaps for preservation of digital length in an 18-month old child. J Hand Surg Eur Vol 2013; 38:89–91.

23. Venkatramani H, Sabapathy SR. A useful technique to maintain the position of the hand following abdominal flap. Indian J Plast Surg 2008;41: 100–1.

Free Skin Flap Coverage of the Upper Extremity

Elizabeth A. King, MD, Kagan Ozer, MD*

KEYWORDS

- Free flap • Upper extremity • Reconstruction • Cutaneous • Coverage • Vascularity

KEY POINTS

- Soft tissue reconstruction for the hand must provide coverage and restore function.
- Early debridement and early flap coverage is important to allow mobilization.
- Many good options for free flap coverage in the upper extremity provide versatility and low donor site morbidity.

INTRODUCTION

In the injured upper extremity, goals of reconstruction encompass not only soft tissue coverage but also restoration of form, function, and sensation. Both patient- and injury-related factors create unique requirements for restoring function and contour of the hand.[1–3] Adequate early debridement and soft tissue coverage allowing early mobilization of the hand are important for improving clinical outcomes.[4]

This article discusses options for free skin flap coverage of the traumatized upper extremity. Early treatment of these injuries often begins with stable bony fixation first, with repair of injured nerves and tendons along with soft tissue coverage.[2] In many cases, free flap coverage should be selected early in the treatment algorithm to achieve a better functional end result.

DEFINITION AND CLASSIFICATION OF SKIN FLAPS

Skin flaps provide cutaneous coverage, and may be local, pedicled, or free. In traumatic hand injuries, availability of local tissue can be scarce, especially if an extensive zone of injury is present, such as in crush injuries or high-pressure injection trauma.[5] This article focuses on free skin flaps for reconstruction, which have their own blood supply and may include skin along with fascia, muscle, bone, or tendon.

Options for skin flap coverage have increased in recent years, leading to some confusion in developing nomenclature. In one proposed classification system, Nakajima and colleagues[6] separate skin flaps into 5 types, which are cutaneous, fasciocutaneous, adipofascial, septocutaneous, and musculocutaneous. Alternately, Cormack and Lamberty[7] divide skin flaps into 3 groups: direct cutaneous, fasciocutaneous, or musculocutaneous flaps. Here the term *fasciocutaneous* is used more broadly to include any or all tissues between the skin and the deep fascia. In general, fasciocutaneous flaps are based on fasciocutaneous perforator vessels, which form a plexus at the level of the deep fascia, and are ideal for covering shallow wounds because they are thin and able to restore both contour and a gliding surface for tendons.[3]

Hallock[8] describes a pattern for complete flap classification based on the "6 Cs" described by Cormack and Lamberty,[7] which includes circulation (blood supply), constituents (composition), contiguity (destination), construction (flow),

Disclosures: Neither the authors nor any immediate family member has any financial relationship to disclose with any financial company or institution directly or indirectly related to the subject of this article.
Department of Orthopaedic Surgery, University of Michigan, 2098 South Main Street, Ann Arbor, MI 48103, USA
* Corresponding author.
E-mail address: kozer@umich.edu

Hand Clin 30 (2014) 201–209
http://dx.doi.org/10.1016/j.hcl.2014.01.003

conditioning (preparation), and conformation (geometry). This system allows for a complete description of any flap, and works toward the goal of developing a common system for communication.[8] This article focuses on free skin flaps, because other types of free flaps are discussed elsewhere in this issue.

FREE VERSUS LOCAL FLAP COVERAGE: INDICATIONS

Local and pedicled flaps work well for coverage of small, isolated defects in the upper extremity, and are technically less demanding than free flaps. However, in mutilating, high-energy injuries, use of a pedicled flap may not be possible because the extensive zone of injury. Free flaps are indicated when local flaps cannot be harvested outside the zone of injury, and also for large soft tissue defects that include exposed bone, tendon, nerves, and vessels.[3] Factors that must be taken into consideration when choosing a flap include the size, shape, location of defect, donor site morbidity, and goals of reconstruction. Soft tissue coverage should be performed as early as possible after adequate debridement.[4,5] If early radical debridement is not possible, then serial debridements should instead be performed before soft tissue coverage.[9]

Free flaps provide the greatest versatility in reconstructive options for the upper extremity. They can include skin, fascia, bone, tendon, or nerve depending on what tissue is needed to cover the defect. Free flaps also have the advantage of bringing their own blood supply along with angiogenic and lymphogenic potential, which improves venous and lymphatic drainage of the traumatized area.[10]

The decision to use a free flap depends on the size and location of the defect, mechanism of injury, exposed structures, structures in need of reconstruction, and the need to restore sensation.[5,9] Goals of free flap reconstruction may include skin coverage, but it can also supply functioning muscle, bone reconstruction, or vascularized nerve grafts if needed. Free flaps have the advantage of providing a large and reliable cutaneous territory with a long vascular pedicle, ensuring that the microvascular anastomosis is well outside the zone of injury.

COMMONLY USED FREE SKIN FLAPS
Venous Free Flaps

Venous flaps are harvested as a skin island with 2 veins. One vein becomes "arterialized" when anastomosed to a recipient artery, and the other vein becomes the flap's outflow. Venous flaps are very thin because they are harvested in the suprafascial plane.[11,12] Arterialized venous flaps can be harvested from the forearm or dorsal foot, and can be useful for resurfacing and revascularizing traumatic defects in the hand, particularly on the dorsal surface.

Woo and colleagues[13] report a 98% success rate in a series of 154 arterialized venous free flaps used for coverage in the upper extremity. The types of flaps in this series included venous skin flaps and tendocutaneous, innervated venous, and conduit venous flaps. The defect sizes ranged from less than 10 cm² in 48 cases (31.0%), between 10 and 25 cm² in 64 cases (42.0%), and greater than 25 cm² in 42 cases (27.0%). Seven cases (4.5%) required emergent return to the operating room: 5 for arterial insufficiency and 2 for venous congestion. Three of these flaps failed.[13] Despite this high success rate, partial flap necrosis is common and can be as high as 5.2% in this series, deserving their description as "reliably unreliable."[2,14]

In a study of 125 flaps for coverage of the dorsum of the hand, Parrett and colleagues[15] compared muscle, fasciocutaneous, fascial, and venous flaps in their aesthetic and functional outcomes; number of secondary procedures; and donor site morbidity. The best aesthetic results were achieved with venous flaps, which were harvested from the volar forearm in the suprafascial plane. The advantages of venous flaps are that they represent a thin and pliable structure, and that they provide a good match for dorsal hand skin without need for later debulking. Furthermore, they do not sacrifice a major artery, and donor site morbidity is minimal. Venous flaps can cover defects up to approximately 40 cm² and are ideal for coverage on the dorsal surface of the hand.[15]

Radial Forearm Flap

The radial forearm flap is a workhorse flap in microsurgical reconstruction, and has remained one of the most popular options because of its thin pliable skin, long pedicle, and large caliber vessel. The radial forearm flap was first described in 1978 by a group of surgeons at the Shenyang Military Hospital, and its use for dorsal hand defects with vascularized tendon transfers was initially described by Reid and Moss[16] in 1983. The radial forearm flap represents a fasciocutaneous flap, and can be used as a reverse pedicle flap for dorsal hand reconstruction or an antegrade pedicle flap for olecranon reconstruction.[14] However, this flap also offers additional versatility, in that it can be harvested with the vascularized palmaris longus, a segment of radius, the antebrachial cutaneous nerve, or the brachioradialis, depending on reconstructive needs.[17] Moreover, unlike other flaps, the radial forearm flap can be used as a flow-through flap to revascularize the hand while providing coverage. Jones and colleagues[18] reported a retrospective analysis of radial forearm flaps for upper extremity coverage, with 57 pedicled and 10 free radial forearm flaps. Indications included dorsal and palmar hand and wrist coverage, and elbow and thumb coverage. The average flap size was 8 × 6 cm, with a 95% success rate and one flap failure caused by inadequate recipient veins. The major disadvantage of the radial forearm flap is its donor site morbidity, which is both aesthetic and functional, because most donor sites will require skin grafting. Patients may also experience dysesthesias in the superficial radial nerve distribution, and the authors recommend ensuring that the superficial radial nerve is covered with forearm skin, and suturing the margins to flexor tendons to reduce these risks. Cold intolerance has also been described at the donor site but was not seen in this series, although authors note that all patients lived in California.[18] At the recipient site, this flap can be bulky because of the subcutaneous fat layer. Furthermore, in men, volar forearm skin may be hairy and therefore not well-suited for coverage of palmar hand defects. Donor site morbidity can be reduced through suprafascial flap harvest and full-thickness grafting at the donor site, as shown in a study of 95 radial forearm flaps by Lutz and colleagues,[19] which reported a 94% rate of complete take of skin grafts and avoidance of impairment in motion and strength in the donor hand. Vascularity in suprafascially harvested radial forearm flaps is nearly identical to that in subfascially harvested radial forearm flaps.[3] The radial forearm flap is also described as a fascial flap that is less bulky and avoids the need for skin grafting at the donor site, but does require grafting at the recipient site.[20]

The use of the radial forearm flap typically involves sacrifice of the radial artery, which requires adequate perfusion to the hand through the ulnar artery. Critical ischemia is not frequently seen in the acute setting because of this collateral flow; however, more recent studies suggest that problems with chronic ischemia may still develop, even in the presence of a normal Allen test designating the presence of a complete arch.[21]

Lateral Arm Flap

The lateral arm flap is based on the posterior radial collateral artery and venae comitantes, supplying a vascular pedicle up to 8 cm in length. Its territory includes the distal half of the lateral arm and proximal third of the dorsolateral forearm, and has the advantage of matching skin color and thickness in the upper extremity.[4] Use of this pedicle does not affect circulation of the hand. The lateral arm flap was initially described by Song and colleagues[22] in 1982, and was clinically introduced by Katsaros and colleagues[23] in 1984. This flap can be harvested as a pure fascial flap or as a composite flap, to include up to 10 cm of humerus or a portion of vascularized triceps if needed.[24,25] The posterior brachii cutaneous nerve can be used if needed for sensate reconstruction.[24] Gosain and colleagues[24] describes a series of 6 patients with vascularized triceps flaps: 3 using triceps muscle and 3 using triceps tendon. None of these patients showed deficits in elbow extension.

Scheker and colleagues[26] described the use of the ipsilateral lateral arm free flap in 29 patients, with a success rate of 96.5% in both elective and emergency reconstruction. In this series, most defects were on the dorsum of the hand. They were able to harvest fascia up to 20 × 14 cm and skin measuring 12 × 6 cm. Donor sites up to 6 cm in width were able to be closed primarily, which is one advantage of this flap. They note that tenderness over the lateral epicondyle can develop if it is not covered with full thickness skin. Additionally, the loss of the lateral cutaneous nerve of the forearm may result in an area of forearm numbness.

Subsequently, Graham and colleagues[27] presented a series of 123 patients with lateral arm flaps, in which 115 flaps were used in upper limb reconstruction, covering an average defect size of 75 cm². The donor site was closed primarily in 62.6% of cases, and the remaining 37.4% of patients required split-thickness skin grafting at the donor site. Complete loss of the flap occurred in 5 patients (4%), and an additional 3 patients (2.6%) experienced partial flap necrosis. The success rate was 97% when reconstruction occurred within 2 weeks of the injury and 82.5% with later reconstruction. Donor site complications in this series included unsatisfactory cosmetic appearance (26.6%), which was a more frequent complaint in women and patients who required split-thickness skin grafting; forearm numbness (58.7%); and lateral epicondylar pain (19.2%). At the recipient site, the most common complication was excessive flap bulk (82.6%), with 15.0% of the total group undergoing further debulking surgery.

Ulusal and colleagues[28] reported a retrospective analysis of 118 lateral arm flaps (104 fasciocutaneous, 6 fascial, and 8 composite), with most indicated for industrial crush injuries. The success rate was 97.5%, with 3 flap failures, 1 for arterial occlusion and 2 for deep infections. In this series, 16.0% of patients required debulking procedures.

Akinci and colleagues[29] described a series of 74 lateral arm flaps for skin defects between 6 × 4 and 20 × 9 cm, with an average flap area of 57.9 cm^2. A total of 5 flaps (7.0%) were lost to venous thrombosis, with 3 occurring in patients with high-voltage electrical burns, which were associated with a higher failure rate, possibly because of endothelial injury.[29] In this series, all patients had forearm numbness that resolved over a 10-month period, and 8.5% underwent thinning and Z-plasty operations. Overall, lateral arm defects provide coverage of moderate-sized defects with low morbidity.

Anterolateral Thigh Flap

The anterolateral thigh flap is based on a descending branch of the lateral femoral circumflex artery. It may be based on either a septocutaneous or musculocutaneous perforator vessel.[30] The vascular pedicle measures up to 15 cm in length, which is excellent for performing arterial anastomosis well outside the zone of injury. The anterolateral thigh flap can be harvested as a fascia-only flap and then skin grafted, or as a suprafascial perforator flap. Like the radial forearm free flap, it can also be used as a flow-through flap to revascularize the hand. Sensate reconstruction can be provided with use of the lateral femoral cutaneous nerve. This flap can also be harvested with vastus lateralis muscle if needed, or with fascia lata that can be used in tendon reconstruction.

The anterolateral thigh flap provides a large and reliable adipocutaneous territory available for soft tissue coverage with minimal donor site morbidity. Donor sites can usually be closed primarily if the width of the harvested flap is less than 8 cm. Because of its structure, this flap is well-suited for resurfacing shallow defects of the upper extremity (**Fig. 1**). The fasciocutaneous version is usually too bulky for hand reconstruction, particularly in obese patients, but can be thinned later to improve the contour.[11] This flap can also be ideal for contracture releases of antecubital fossa and axilla after burn injuries (**Fig. 2**).

Wang and colleagues[30] reported a retrospective analysis of 15 patients who underwent upper extremity reconstruction using the anterolateral thigh flap. The size of the flap ranged from 64 to 450 cm^2, with an average area of 159 cm^2. The donor site closed primarily in 8 patients (53%) with a skin graft required in 7 patients (47%). The overall flap survival rate was 93%, with one patient experiencing complete flap

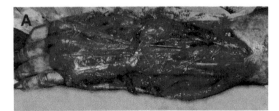
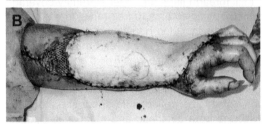
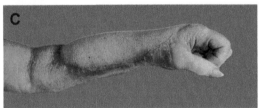
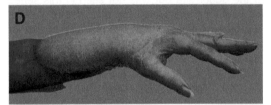
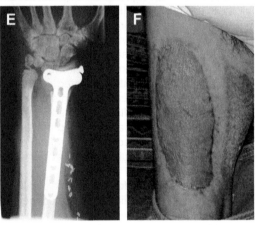

Fig. 1. Right hand–dominant woman aged 65 years involved in a motor vehicle rollover accident who sustained an isolated open distal radius and ulna fracture with significant soft tissue loss on the dorsal aspect of her left hand and forearm (*A*). After initial debridement and open reduction and internal fixation of her fractures, she had an anterolateral thigh free flap for soft tissue reconstruction (*B*). Her functional status 6 months after the surgery is shown (*C–E*). The donor site was primarily skin grafted at the time of the initial reconstruction (*F*).

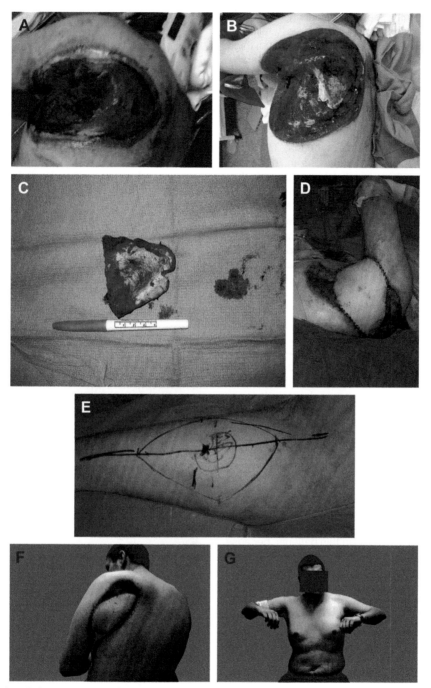

Fig. 2. Right hand–dominant man aged 26 years involved in a motor vehicle accident who sustained a full-thickness burn on the left axilla. (*A*) He had a large soft tissue defect after serial debridements of the skin, scapula, and latissimus dorsi (*B, C*). Ipsilateral anterolateral thigh flap was chosen for reconstruction of the defect because of its large size (*D, E*). Six months after the surgery, he was able to abduct his shoulder up to 90° without pain (*F, G*). Further treatment was planned for the repair of a rotator cuff.

loss because of wound infection and 2 patients requiring debridement of partial necrosis. One patient experienced wound breakdown at the donor site. Advantages of the anterolateral thigh flap include a large surface area, a long vascular pedicle, and the ability to thin the flap for better contour. Additionally, the procedure can be performed with the patient supine, allowing simultaneous donor site harvest and recipient site preparation.

In a prospective series evaluating donor site morbidity, Hanasono and colleagues[31] followed 220 patients who underwent anterolateral thigh flap harvest over a 3-year period. The average flap width was 7.8 cm and the average length was 19.2 cm. Primary closure of the donor site was possible in 85% of patients, with 15% requiring skin grafting. They found that 84% of patients experienced numbness in the lateral femoral cutaneous nerve distribution. The most common donor site complications in this series were seroma (5%), wound dehiscence (2%), hematoma (1%), infection (1%), neuroma (1%), and partial skin graft loss (1%).[31]

Donor site morbidity is relatively low. However, the donor site scar may be unsightly, especially in patients with a high body mass index. Overall, the anterolateral thigh flap works well for upper extremity reconstruction because of the large amount of skin available, its versatility, and the reliability of the flap.

Thoracodorsal Artery Flap

The thoracodorsal artery flap is based on a perforator from the descending branch of the thoracodorsal artery, which has a large cutaneous vascular territory and may be harvested with minimal donor site morbidity. The thoracodorsal artery supplies the latissimus dorsi muscle with perforators to the skin. This flap was originally described in 1995 by Angrigiani and colleagues[32] as a series of 5 cases based on the perforators coming through the latissimus dorsi muscle, and was proposed as a better choice for reconstruction of the hand. The thoracodorsal artery flap is ideal for resurfacing shallow defects in thin patients, because it can be thinned if necessary between deep and superficial adipose layers. Depending on reconstructive needs, this flap can be combined with a portion of latissimus dorsi muscle, serratus muscle, or serratus fascia, or a segment of scapula (**Fig. 3**).[33,34]

Case series' specifically reporting results of the thoracodorsal artery perforator flap are limited because latissimus dorsi muscle is often included in the flap. Chen and colleagues[35] described the use of a thoracodorsal artery flap for distal limb reconstruction in 12 cases: 3 hands, 2 forearms, and 7 feet. Flap sizes ranged from 5 × 3 to 17 × 9 cm, and all were based on a single perforator. All donor sites were closed primarily. One flap developed venous congestion and partial necrosis, but no complete flap losses occurred. Advantages of this flap include minimal donor site morbidity, because muscle function is preserved. However, this flap requires meticulous intramuscular

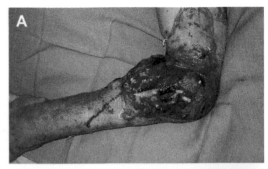
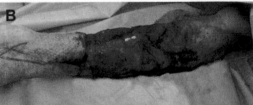
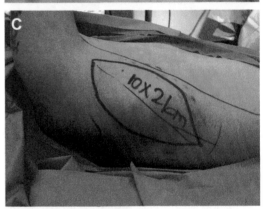
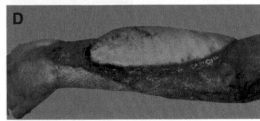

Fig. 3. Right hand–dominant woman aged 22 years with a history of narcotic drug presented to the emergency room with a draining wound because of frequent "skin popping" (*A*). After serial debridements, she had an extensive area of skin and muscle loss on the extensor surface of the forearm (*B*). A latissimus dorsi flap along with a large skin paddle was designed to cover the defect (*C*). Final result 3 months after the surgery is shown (*D*).

dissection of the perforator back to the thoracodorsal artery to get a suitable pedicle length and vessel diameter, which can prolong surgery time.

In another series, Sever and colleagues[36] described the use of the thoracodorsal artery perforator fasciocutaneous flap in 13 patients. In this series, 4 patients had antecubital burn contractures, 3 had axillary burn contractures, 3 had axillary reconstruction for recurrent hidradenitis, and 2 had crush injuries. The donor site was closed primarily in all cases. Transient venous congestion occurred in 2 patients, and donor site seroma occurred in 1 patient.

Scapular-Parascapular Flap

The scapular flap is based on the transverse cutaneous scapular branch of the circumflex scapular artery, whereas the parascapular flap is based on the vertical parascapular branch of the circumflex scapular artery after it traverses the triangular space. Both provide a large vascular territory with a long pedicle that is capable of covering large defects.[5] Both scapular and parascapular flaps can be combined with latissimus dorsi or serratus muscle, if needed. They can also be harvested with a vascularized segment of bone from the lateral border of the scapula for bony reconstruction. This flap is well-suited for releasing contractures around the axillary region.[37]

Hashmi[38] described 11 free scapular flaps used for coverage of large upper extremity defects, averaging 18×11 cm. Upper extremity defects resulted from road traffic accidents (n = 8), bomb blasts (n = 2), and industrial injury (n = 1). The donor site was closed primarily in all cases. Outcomes were evaluated based on cosmetic appearance, coverage of defect, return to daily activities, and range of motion over joints, which was graded "excellent" in 7 cases and "good" in the remaining 4. In another series of 12 extremity reconstructions using free scapular fascial flaps, only one flap was lost because of vascular thrombosis, with an average flap size of 197 cm^2, and the largest around 250 cm^2.[39]

Izadi and colleagues[40] provided a retrospective analysis of 45 free fasciocutaneous flaps of the subscapular axis, which included scapular, parascapular, and thoracodorsal artery perforator flaps. All donor sites were closed primarily with minimal donor site morbidity, and all flaps in this series survived. Donor site morbidity was evaluated objectively with the Medical Research Council (MRC) score; Vancouver Scar Scale; and disability of arm, shoulder, and hand questionnaire (DASH) scores. No difference in power on the donor shoulder side was observed. Authors reported minimal donor site morbidity based on the scar score and the DASH scores.[40] Klinkenberg and colleagues[41] performed a retrospective analysis of 60 patients who underwent free flap reconstruction of the upper extremity, including 20 parascapular flaps, 20 anterolateral thigh flaps, and 20 lateral arm flaps. Their focus was on comparing donor site morbidity and aesthetic and functional outcomes based on the DASH score, Lower Extremity Functional Scale, and SF-36. All of these scores showed no significant differences. However, when comparing overall donor site complication rates (including seroma, hematoma, dehiscence, and altered sensation), the lowest donor site morbidity and highest patient satisfaction outcomes were in the parascapular flap group.[41]

Temporoparietal Fascia Flap

The temporoparietal fascia is a superior extension of the superficial musculoaponeurotic system, and the temporoparietal fascia flap is based on the superficial temporal artery and vein. The flap is ultrathin and highly vascular, and provides a gliding surface that is well-suited for reconstruction of the hand.[42] It has a robust pedicle but requires a meticulous dissection, during which care must be taken to avoid injuring the auriculotemporal nerve. It is harvested as a fascial flap only, which requires skin grafting at the recipient site. The donor site is closed primarily and well hidden within the hairline, which provides a cosmetic advantage.

Carty and colleagues[43] recently reported their experience in covering traumatic injuries to the dorsum of the hand. They reported on 60 fascial flaps, 35 of which were temporoparietal flaps. All flaps in their series survived with excellent aesthetic and functional outcome, with no tendon adhesions reported. The fascial strength, thinness, and pliability of this flap provide excellent coverage for the dorsum of the hand or palmar surfaces. The flap can be used to cover defects up to 14×12 cm in the hand or fingers.[44] It can be performed as a single-stage coverage that has the advantage of providing a surface that does not adhere to underlying nerve or require tendon, vascular, or skeletal repairs.

Kruavit and Visuthikosol[45] described use of the temporoparietal fascia flap for correction of first web space atrophy in a series of 13 patients with ulnar nerve palsy. Of these patients, 10 had ulnar nerve injuries and 3 had leprosy. Defect sizes in the first web space varied from 4×5 to 6×8 cm, and the temporoparietal fascia free flap was successfully used to fill the area in all cases. No resorption was seen at follow-up, and all patients were satisfied with the postoperative results.

SUMMARY

Successful soft tissue reconstruction of the upper extremity must provide stable coverage and restore function to the injured hand. The hand does not tolerate prolonged immobilization, because joint stiffness and tendon adhesions can severely limit future function. To ensure the best possible outcome after traumatic upper extremity injuries, early radical debridement and early flap coverage that restores all missing tissue components is critical to allow early mobilization. Free flaps provide extraordinary versatility in reconstructing defects of soft tissue, muscle, tendon, and bone. Free flaps can also provide obliteration of dead space in complex 3-dimensional defects, with restoration of normal contour and coverage of exposed vital structures, while providing a smooth tendon gliding surface. Further research is needed to address functional outcomes for specific flaps to continue to guide treatment of these challenging injuries.

REFERENCES

1. Kutz JA, Copit SE, Moore JH Jr. Soft tissue reconstruction of the upper extremity. Operat Tech Orthop 1997;7(2):100–6.
2. Neumeister M, Hegge T, Amalfi A, et al. The reconstruction of the mutilated hand. Semin Plast Surg 2010;24(1):77–102.
3. Saint-Cyr M, Gupta A. Indications and selection of free flaps for soft tissue coverage of the upper extremity. Hand Clin 2007;23(1):37–48.
4. Scheker LR, Ahmed O. Radical debridement, free flap coverage, and immediate reconstruction of the upper extremity. Hand Clin 2007;23(1):23–36.
5. Giessler GA, Erdmann D, Germann G. Soft tissue coverage in devastating hand injuries. Hand Clinics 2003;19(1):63–71.
6. Nakajima H, Fujino T, Adachi S. A new concept of vascular supply to the skin and classification of skin flaps according to their vascularization. Ann Plast Surg 1986;16(1):1–19.
7. Cormack GC, Lamberty BG. The arterial anatomy of skin flaps. 2nd edition. Edinburg (TX): Churchill Livingston; 1994.
8. Hallock GG. The complete classification of flaps. Microsurgery 2004;24(3):157–61.
9. Gupta A, Shatford RA, Wolff TW, et al. Treatment of the severely injured upper extremity. Instr Course Lect 2000;49:377–96.
10. Slavin SA, Upton J, Kaplan WD, et al. An investigation of lymphatic function following free-tissue transfer. Plast Reconstr Surg 1997;99(3):730–41 [discussion: 742–3].
11. Friedrich JB, Katolik LI, Vedder NB. Soft tissue reconstruction of the hand. J Hand Surg Am 2009; 34(6):1148–55.
12. Kong BS, Kim YJ, Suh YS, et al. Finger soft tissue reconstruction using arterialized venous free flaps having 2 parallel veins. J Hand Surg Am 2008; 33(10):1802–6.
13. Woo SH, Kim KC, Lee GJ, et al. A retrospective analysis of 154 arterialized venous flaps for hand reconstruction: an 11-year experience. Plast Reconstr Surg 2007;119(6):1823–38.
14. Soutar DS, Tanner NS. The radial forearm flap in the management of soft tissue injuries of the hand. Br J Plast Surg 1984;37(1):18–26.
15. Parrett BM, Bou-Merhi JS, Buntic RF, et al. Refining outcomes in dorsal hand coverage: consideration of aesthetics and donor-site morbidity. Plast Reconstr Surg 2010;126(5):1630–8.
16. Reid CD, Moss LH. One-stage flap repair with vascularised tendon grafts in a dorsal hand injury using the "Chinese" forearm flap. Br J Plast Surg 1983; 36(4):473–9.
17. Foucher G, van Genechten F, Merle N, et al. A compound radial artery forearm flap in hand surgery: an original modification of the Chinese forearm flap. Br J Plast Surg 1984;37(2):139–48.
18. Jones NF, Jarrahy R, Kaufman MR. Pedicled and free radial forearm flaps for reconstruction of the elbow, wrist, and hand. Plast Reconstr Surg 2008; 121(3):887–98.
19. Lutz BS, Wei FC, Chang SC, et al. Donor site morbidity after suprafascial elevation of the radial forearm flap: a prospective study in 95 consecutive cases. Plast Reconstr Surg 1999;103(1):132–7.
20. Friedrich JB, Pederson WC, Bishop AT, et al. New workhorse flaps in hand reconstruction. Hand (N Y) 2012;7(1):45–54.
21. Higgins JP. A reassessment of the role of the radial forearm flap in upper extremity reconstruction. J Hand Surg Am 2011;36(7):1237–40.
22. Song R, Song Y, Yu Y, et al. The upper arm free flap. Clin Plast Surg 1982;9(1):27–35.
23. Katsaros J, Schusterman M, Beppu M, et al. The lateral upper arm flap: anatomy and clinical applications. Ann Plast Surg 1984;12(6):489–500.
24. Gosain AK, Matloub HS, Sanger JR. The composite lateral arm free flap: vascular relationship to triceps tendon and muscle. Ann Plast Surg 1992;29(6):496–507.
25. Chen HC, Buchman MT, Wei FC. Free flaps for soft tissue coverage in the hand and fingers. Hand Clin 1999;15(4):541–54.
26. Scheker LR, Kleinert HE, Hanel DP. Lateral arm composite tissue transfer to ipsilateral hand defects. J Hand Surg Am 1987;12(5 Part 1):665–72.
27. Graham B, Adkins P, Scheker LR. Complications and morbidity of the donor and recipient sites in 123 lateral arm flaps. J Hand Surg Br 1992;17(2):189–92.
28. Ulusal BG, Lin YT, Ulusal AE, et al. Free lateral arm flap for 1-stage reconstruction of soft tissue and composite defects of the hand: a retrospective analysis of 118 cases. Ann Plast Surg 2007;58(2):173–8.
29. Akinci M, Ay S, Kamiloglu S, et al. Lateral arm free flaps in the defects of the upper extremity—a review of 72 cases. Hand Surg 2005;10(2–3):177–85.

30. Wang HT, Fletcher JW, Erdmann D, et al. Use of the anterolateral thigh free flap for upper-extremity reconstruction. J Hand Surg Am 2005;30(4):859–64.

31. Hanasono MM, Skoracki RJ, Yu P. A prospective study of donor-site morbidity after anterolateral thigh fasciocutaneous and myocutaneous free flap harvest in 220 patients. Plast Reconstr Surg 2010; 125(1):209–14.

32. Angrigiani C, Grilli D, Siebert J. Latissimus dorsi musculocutaneous flap without muscle. Plast Reconstr Surg 1995;96(7):1608–14.

33. Bidros RS, Metzinger SE, Guerra AB. The thoracodorsal artery perforator-scapular osteocutaneous (TDAP-SOC) flap for reconstruction of palatal and maxillary defects. Ann Plast Surg 2005;54(1):59–65.

34. Van Landuyt K, Hamdi M, Blondeel P, et al. The compound thoracodorsal perforator flap in the treatment of combined soft-tissue defects of sole and dorsum of the foot. Br J Plast Surg 2005;58(3):371–8.

35. Chen SL, Chen TM, Wang HJ. Free thoracodorsal artery perforator flap in extremity reconstruction: 12 cases. Br J Plast Surg 2004;57(6):525–30.

36. Sever C, Uygur F, Kulahci Y, et al. Thoracodorsal artery perforator fasciocutaneous flap: a versatile alternative for coverage of various soft tissue defects. Indian J Plast Surg 2012;45(3):478–84.

37. Romana MC, Goubier JN, Gilbert A, et al. Coverage of large skin defects of the pediatric upper extremity. Hand Clin 2000;16(4):563–71.

38. Hashmi PM. Free scapular flap for reconstruction of upper extremity defects. J Coll Physicians Surg Pak 2004;14(8):485–8.

39. Datiashvili RO, Yueh JH. Management of complicated wounds of the extremities with scapular fascial free flaps. J Reconstr Microsurg 2012;28(8): 521–8.

40. Izadi D, Paget JT, Haj-Basheer M, et al. Fasciocutaneous flaps of the subscapular artery axis to reconstruct large extremity defects. J Plast Reconstr Aesthet Surg 2012;65(10):1357–62.

41. Klinkenberg M, Fischer S, Kremer T, et al. Comparison of anterolateral thigh, lateral arm, and parascapular free flaps with regard to donor-site morbidity and aesthetic and functional outcomes. Plast Reconstr Surg 2013;131(2):293–302.

42. Brent B, Upton J, Acland RD, et al. Experience with the temporoparietal fascial free flap. Plast Reconstr Surg 1985;76(2):177–88.

43. Carty MJ, Taghinia A, Upton J. Fascial flap reconstruction of the hand: a single surgeon's 30-year experience. Plast Reconstr Surg 2010;125(3): 953–62.

44. Upton J, Rogers C, Durham-Smith G, et al. Clinical applications of free temporoparietal flaps in hand reconstruction. J Hand Surg Am 1986;11(4):475–83.

45. Kruavit A, Visuthikosol V. Temporoparietal fascial free flap for correction of first web space atrophy. Microsurgery 2010;30(1):8–12.

Refinements and Secondary Surgery After Flap Reconstruction of the Traumatized Hand

Grace J. Chiou, MD[a,b], James Chang, MD[a,c],*

KEYWORDS

- Traumatized hand • Flap reconstruction • Secondary flap elevation • Secondary procedures
- Functional refinements

KEY POINTS

- The need for refinement and secondary surgery should be taken into consideration during the initial flap selection process.
- Muscle flaps may achieve better contour than bulky fasciocutaneous flaps.
- Fasciocutaneous flaps permit easier secondary flap elevation, and thereby provide versatile soft tissue coverage in the setting of anticipated secondary reconstruction of the traumatized hand.
- The need for secondary procedures can be classified based on the type of tissue that requires revision after initial reconstruction.

INTRODUCTION

Secondary refinements after flap reconstruction of the traumatized hand depend on the type of flap used during primary reconstruction, in addition to the functional and aesthetic problems subsequently encountered. Achieving optimal hand function is the ultimate goal after encountering mutilating trauma to the hand. Several prerequisites should be fulfilled in order to attain this goal. Such requirements include the acquisition of adaptable and ample soft tissue coverage, bony stabilization, adequate joint mobility, smooth-gliding tendons, functional muscle strength, and restoration of sensation.[1]

FLAP RECONSTRUCTION

An anticipatory operative plan is fundamental to ensuring optimal soft tissue coverage of the hand during the process of establishing functional restoration, while taking care to minimize donor-site morbidity. Multiple factors contribute to flap selection. Most of these factors are attributed to matching the characteristics of the original defect: size, contour, location, and quality of tissues missing from the defect. The most common currently used flaps for reconstruction of the traumatized hand include musculocutaneous, muscle, fasciocutaneous, and fascial flaps.

Musculocutaneous and Muscle Flaps

Musculocutaneous and muscle flaps can be obtained from muscles such as the latissimus dorsi, rectus abdominis, serratus anterior, and gracilis. Most of these flaps are used as muscle-only flaps, and are subsequently covered with skin graft. Superiority of soft tissue coverage with a muscle-only

Disclosures: None.
[a] Division of Plastic and Reconstructive Surgery, Stanford University Medical Center, 770 Welch Road, Suite 400, Stanford, CA 94304, USA; [b] VA Palo Alto Division of Plastic and Reconstructive Surgery, VA Palo Alto, 3801 Miranda Avenue, Building 100, Room F4-241, Palo Alto, CA 94304, USA; [c] Plastic and Hand Surgery Laboratory, Veterans Affairs Palo Alto Health Care System, 3801 Miranda Avenue, Palo Alto, CA 94304, USA
* Corresponding author. Division of Plastic and Reconstructive Surgery, Stanford University Medical Center, 770 Welch Road, Suite 400, Stanford, CA 94304.
E-mail address: jameschang@stanford.edu

Hand Clin 30 (2014) 211–223
http://dx.doi.org/10.1016/j.hcl.2014.01.004

flap versus a myocutaneous flap remains equivocal.[2] Advantages of these flaps include their ranges in dimensions, ability to eliminate dead space in sizable defects, and rich blood supply. An additional benefit of these musculocutaneous and muscle flaps is their suitability for antibiotic delivery. For this reason, they have been the flaps of choice in defects complicated by extensive contamination, in addition to osteomyelitis.[3] These flaps also atrophy after denervation, and they contour well after their initial bulky size (**Fig. 1**). Despite these benefits, these flaps have some disadvantages. The color mismatch and appearance of the overlying skin graft may cause an unappealing appearance. If revision is required, these flaps are difficult to debulk and cannot be split into layers to allow tunneling of tendons or nerves. In addition, the donor site loses motor function.

Fasciocutaneous Flaps

Common fasciocutaneous flaps include the lateral arm, anterolateral thigh (**Box 1**), radial forearm, scapula, and parascapular flaps. Their pliable nature allows straightforward flap re-elevation, in addition to flexible contouring to the size and shape of the original wound. Although these flaps offer increased flexibility, the amount of donor tissue is limited by the ability to achieve primary

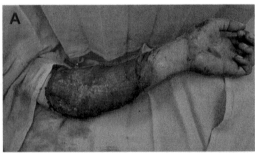

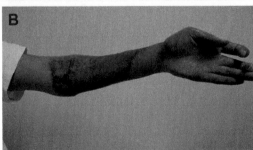

Fig. 1. (*A*) Initial reconstruction of a large defect over the antecubital fossa extending distally to the midforearm, with a latissimus dorsi muscle flap. (*B*) The same defect 6 months from the original flap reconstruction. The bulkiness of the original flap has atrophied, and now shows good contour.

> **Box 1**
> **Latest advances: outcomes of the anterolateral thigh flap**
>
> The anterolateral thigh flap offers versatility in size and shape. Flap thickness may easily be adjusted to match the needs of the soft tissue defect, including additional harvest of the tensor fasciae latae to reconstruct tendon and soft tissue deficiencies simultaneously. In the past, concern about the anatomic variability of its cutaneous blood supply limited the flap's use.[3] However, Wei and colleagues' study of 672 anterolateral thigh flaps showed that these flaps could be harvested without regard for the origin of the cutaneous blood supply (ie, septocutaneous or musculocutaneous). Furthermore, the study showed a 1.79% total and 2.53% partial flap failure rate. Given these results, Wei and colleagues[4] concluded that the anterolateral flap may be substituted for almost any flap required in most soft tissue reconstructions.

closure of the donor defect. In addition, their advantageous thin, and pliable characteristics may not be found in obese patients, given these patients' greater flap thickness.[3] Bulky fasciocutaneous flaps have a biscuit appearance that may be difficult to revise (**Fig. 2**).

Fascial Flaps

Common fascial flaps include temporoparietal, anterolateral thigh, radial forearm (**Fig. 3**), and lateral arm flaps. These flaps are a variant of the fasciocutaneous flaps, harvested by leaving the overlying skin intact. These flaps provide even more flexibility than fasciocutaneous flaps, because they are extremely thin. Fascial flaps are excellent for coverage of exposed tendons. These tendons

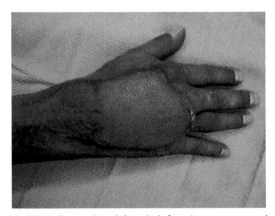

Fig. 2. A large dorsal hand defect is reconstructed with a radial forearm fasciocutaneous flap, in addition to a skin graft for proximal coverage. The radial forearm flap has a bulky appearance.

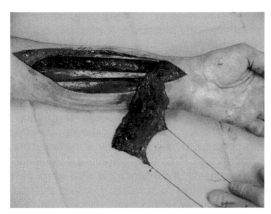

Fig. 3. An intraoperative view after harvest of a radial forearm fascial flap.

may be embedded within fascial flaps, which provide smooth surfaces on which the tendons can enjoy full mobility. For this reason, fascial flaps serve as optimal coverage for dorsal hand defects. One disadvantage of this flap is the need for a second donor site, because these flaps require skin graft coverage.[3]

Flap Selection

A final consideration in flap selection should be the anticipated need for secondary reconstruction. As such, the safety and fluidity of flap re-elevation and flap revision should contribute to the decision-making process. Studies have shown that musculocutaneous, muscle, and fasciocutaneous flaps provide comparable effective coverage of soft tissue defects. Yazar and colleagues compared variables such as rates of flap survival, postoperative infection, chronic osteomyelitis, primary and overall bone union, and postoperative functional status in 147 patients receiving either a free muscle flap or a free fasciocutaneous flap for soft tissue reconstruction of an open, distal tibial fracture. No statistically significant differences were found among all variables studied.[4] Despite equal functional outcomes, fasciocutaneous flaps offer several advantages compared with musculocutaneous and muscle flaps when secondary operations are expected.[5] Fasciocutaneous flaps contain a dermal plexus layer, which provides a safe plane of dissection.[6] Unlike musculocutaneous and muscle flaps, these flaps become less dependent on their primary pedicle with increased time from the initial flap reconstruction. This independence allows fasciocutaneous flaps to be restructured with decreased regard for damaging the vascular supply.[7] Their pliable nature also limits the scarring and contractures that their muscle counterparts have the propensity to form. For

these reasons, fasciocutaneous flaps are ideal when considering possible flap re-elevation. In addition, these flaps offer increased flexibility with contouring during secondary flap revisions. Furthermore, they offer less donor-site morbidity than musculocutaneous and muscle flaps because their donor-site motor function remains intact.[3] As a result of these advantages, the fasciocutaneous flap is the optimal choice for initial soft tissue reconstruction when secondary procedures are foreseen.

REFINEMENTS AND SECONDARY PROCEDURES

The primary goal of secondary operation is to restore optimal hand function. The need for secondary procedures can be classified based on the type of problem the hand and upper extremity may encounter after the initial reconstruction: (1) nonunion, malunion; (2) joint stiffness; (3) tendon adhesions, tendon deficiency; (4) motor and/or sensory nerve deficits, neuroma pain; (5) web space contracture and bulky appearance. Increased severity of structural damage at initial injury increases the likelihood that a patient will require a secondary procedure.[1]

Secondary flap elevation and revision may be undertaken as early as 6 weeks after the initial flap reconstruction.[3] However, in general, secondary procedures should be delayed until soft tissue equilibrium has been achieved, which usually requires 3 to 6 months. During this time period, appropriate soft tissue coverage, tissue vascularity, and bony restoration must be achieved. Bone or nerve grafting are exclusions to these criteria, because patients should undergo these procedures promptly.[8] As a rule, secondary operations necessitating postoperative hand immobilization should be performed before those requiring early physical rehabilitation. Thus, procedures such as bony fixation, tendon reconstruction, and nerve grafting should take place before procedures releasing joint capsules and tendon adhesions.[1] The following details, in order of surgical encounter, the most common problems that may arise in the traumatized hand after initial reconstruction.

Secondary Bone Procedures

The likelihood of bony malunion or nonunion increases with factors such as increased severity of the original trauma, smoking, and initial inadequate treatment. These complications are typically diagnosed by symptoms, physical examination, and radiographic imaging about 4 to 8 weeks after the injury for malunion, and approximately 4 months after the injury for nonunion (**Fig. 4**).[9] Malunion and nonunion that are functionally detrimental often mandate secondary operations. These operations should be performed during the initial stages of secondary reconstruction because they require postoperative immobilization.

Malunion

Malunion complications are common, especially among phalangeal fractures. Buchler and colleagues[10] described the phalangeal malunion distribution among 59 fractures to be 7%, 24%, and 69% in the distal, middle, and proximal phalanges, respectively. Malunion usually occurs secondary to primary bone misalignment, inadequate postsurgical stabilization, repeated trauma, and/or osseous resorption. As a result, patients may experience pain, decreased pinch and grip strength, digital scissoring, and digital shortening.[11,12] Corrective osteotomies are often the treatment of choice. Extra-articular malunions may be classified as angular or rotational. Optimal correction for angular deformities occurs at the point of malunion. These deformities may be managed with either an opening or a closing wedge osteotomy, in addition to internal fixation.

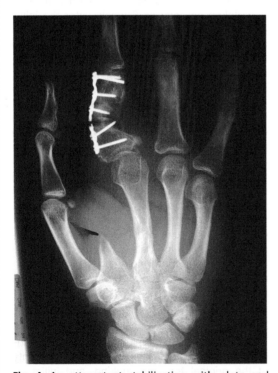

Fig. 4. An attempt at stabilization with plate and screw fixation of a midshaft fracture to the proximal phalanx has been complicated by bony nonunion, as shown by this radiograph. Note breakage of the plate over time.

In general, closing wedge osteotomies are straightforward procedures, whereas opening wedge osteotomies often require more complex steps, such as insertion of an intercalated bone graft. Rotational deformities may be treated with either transverse or step-cut, derotational osteotomies, in addition to rigid fixation. This method allows stabilization and immediate rehabilitation. If intra-articular malunion is present, either an intra-articular or extra-articular osteotomy may be performed.[13] Overall, corrective osteotomies for phalangeal and metacarpal malunions have shown excellent outcomes. Buchler and colleagues[10] achieved full correction in 76% of 59 phalangeal osteotomies, without complications of delayed union or nonunion. In addition, van der Lei and colleagues[11] achieved full correction in 87%, and bony union in 100% of 15 patients treated with corrective osteotomies for both phalangeal and metacarpal fractures.

Nonunion

Bony nonunion in the hand is a rare occurrence. Barton's[14] and Borgeskov's[15] articles report a 0.7% incidence of nonunions occurring in 148 phalangeal fractures and a 0.2% incidence in 485 phalangeal and metacarpal fractures, respectively.[14,15] Nonunion usually occurs as a result of concomitant neurovascular injury on initial trauma, bony deficiency, and/or infection.[16] Operative management for bony nonunion is encouraged because it decreases the time of immobilization, thereby expediting physical rehabilitation and improving functional results of the hand.[12] Hypertrophic nonunion develops when ossification surrounds the site of fragmentation, but excludes the region of nonunion. This type of nonunion is usually secondary to mechanical strain. The usual treatment of hypertrophic nonunion involves mechanical stabilization at the point of nonunion. Atrophic nonunion usually results from impaired biological healing.[17] In these cases, metabolic conditions that could potentially preclude bony formation should be excluded. Atrophic nonunion is managed by improving the blood supply with resection of the nonunion site. If this results in unsatisfactory digital shortening, a bone graft may be applied.[13,16]

Autografts are the optimal choice in bony reconstruction. These bone grafts may be cancellous or corticocancellous. Cancellous bone promotes increased osteogenesis, whereas cortical bone offers more structural stability. Furthermore, these bone grafts may be harvested as nonvascularized or vascularized grafts. Conventional, or nonvascularized, bone graft incorporation is achieved via creeping substitution, which takes approximately

6 months to a year to reach maximal recovery. These grafts may be harvested from locations such as the metacarpals, radius, ulna, and iliac crest. Two main advantages of conventional bone grafts are their accessibility for harvest and their limited donor-site morbidity. However, a disadvantage of the conventional bone graft is its paucity of perfusion during the initial period.[18] Thus, for bony defects less than 6 cm with a well-vascularized bed, no evidence of infection, and good soft tissue coverage, conventional bone grafts should be used. In contrast, for defects greater than 6 cm, vascularized bone grafts should be considered. In addition, bone injuries complicated by factors such as avascular necrosis, composite tissue loss, and physeal arrest should consider the use of these vascularized grafts. Vascularized bone grafts allow the transfer of viable bone tissue, promoting superior cell survival, increased repair strength, and decreased frequency of stress fractures compared with conventional bone grafts. These grafts may be harvested from sites such as the fibula, iliac crest, distal radius, and medial femoral condyle (**Box 2**). Despite the benefits of the immediate, viable tissue they provide for reconstruction, harvesting vascularized bone grafts may be time consuming and may increase the risk of donor-site morbidity compared with conventional bone grafts.[19]

The aforementioned modes of management for bony nonunion have resulted in favorable outcomes. Using a combination of plate fixation, Kirschner wire fixation, excision of the nonunion site, and bone graft to treat 18 phalangeal and metacarpal nonunions of various severities, Jupiter and colleagues[20] showed a 100% success rate in achieving bony union.

Box 2
Latest advances: the medial femoral condyle flap

For recalcitrant nonunions with defects less than 6 cm, an ideal free vascularized bone graft has been difficult to identify. The more commonly used iliac crest and fibula flaps have seen a 12% and 16% flap failure rate, respectively, in addition to suboptimal size matching to the original defect site.[21] Choudry and colleagues[22] proposed the usage of the medial femoral condyle flap because this flap offers flexibility in both size and bony contouring secondary to its periosteal pliability. In their study of 12 bony nonunions that underwent reconstruction with a medial femoral condyle flap, 75% achieved primary bony union over an average of 3.8 months; only 1 of the flaps failed as a result of arterial thrombosis.

Secondary Joint Procedures

Joint stiffness is a common problem that may arise as a result of trauma to the hand. Because the hand and fingers rely on joints for full mobility in range-of-motion activities, joint stiffness may limit hand function, hindering optimal recovery. Two potential causes of joint stiffness are joint contractures and posttraumatic arthroses.

Joint stiffness secondary to joint contracture

Joint contractures usually occur as a result of persistent fluid, either from proteinaceous and macrophage-filled fluid or hematoma, expanding the synovial space. This expansion causes contraction of the joint capsular structures and collateral ligaments.[23] The most common sites of joint contracture after hand trauma are the phalangeal joints.[8] The treatment of choice is usually a capsulotomy, and is most common to the management of proximal interphalangeal (PIP) joints and metacarpophalangeal (MCP) joints, because distal interphalangeal (DIP) joints often do not improve after capsulotomy.[12] Management of extension contractures necessitates tenolysis of the extensor mechanism and release of the dorsal joint capsule. Severe contractures may additionally require release of the transverse retinacular ligament, the volar plate checkrein ligaments, and the accessory radial and ulnar collateral ligaments. After surgery, splints should be applied until stable range of motion is achieved. This level of function is typically attained by 2 to 3 months.[23] Overall, capsulotomy has proved to be an effective treatment of joint contractures, as shown by Young and colleagues'[24] study of 135 PIP and MCP joint contractures. Among the PIP joints undergoing capsulotomies, 63% achieved greater than a 30° arc of motion, and, among the MCP joints, 68% achieved greater than a 30° arc of motion.

Joint stiffness secondary to posttraumatic arthrosis

Posttraumatic arthrosis is another cause of joint stiffness. Often, these are treated with either arthrodesis or amputation, because the bone stock is usually lacking and the supporting soft tissue coverage is in marked disequilibrium. Although motion is sacrificed, arthrodesis provides painless joint stability. The DIP and PIP joints are the most common phalangeal joints that undergo this procedure. The MCP joint should be spared whenever possible, because this joint is a main contributor to functional arc of motion.[25] Only after all conservative attempts have failed to restore painless and effective joint motion should arthrodesis be considered. Two important elements in performing an arthrodesis include good surface preparation and fixation. The bone ends should be contoured such that cancellous-to-cancellous bone apposition is satisfactory. Fixation can then be performed using various methods including Kirschner wires, intraosseous wires, screws, plates, or external fixation. Once fixation is achieved, the joint is immobilized until radiographic evidence of bony union is visualized. The most common complication observed after undergoing arthrodesis is nonunion. Of 50 posttraumatic DIP joint arthrodeses studied by Stern and Fulton,[26] 10% were complicated by nonunion and 2% by malunion, and, of 53 posttraumatic PIP joint arthrodesis studied by Leibovic and Strickland,[27] 9% were complicated by nonunion and 2% by malunion.

When adequate bone stock is present and healthy soft tissue equilibrium has been achieved, arthroplasty should sometimes be considered. The complexity of arthroplasty procedures spans a wide range (eg, silicone elastomer arthroplasty, surface replacement arthroplasty, pyrocarbon arthroplasty), depending on the severity of the initial trauma to the surrounding structures and the comfort of the surgeon with the procedure (**Box 3**).[23]

Secondary Tendon Procedures

Flexor tendon injury and reconstruction

Secondary tendon procedures are performed when tendon adhesions severely limiting digital

---

> **Box 3**
> **Latest advances: pyrocarbon arthroplasty**
>
> In joint arthroplasty, pyrocarbon implants have recently been introduced as a more biologically and anatomically compatible alternative to silicone implants. The properties of pyrocarbon include resistance to wear, in addition to an elastic modulus comparable with that of cortical bone; these characteristics contribute to the implant's durability.[28] Studies have shown good overall patient satisfaction. In McGuire and colleagues'[29] study of 57 PIP joints that underwent pyrocarbon arthroplasty, 88% experienced pain relief, despite a high complication rate of ~42%; these complications included joint squeaking, dislocations, stiffness, and fractures at the implant insertion site.[30] Regardless of these good outcomes in pain relief, Chan and colleagues'[31] literature review revealed no clear advantage in functional outcomes of pyrocarbon arthroplasty compared with silicone implants in 1882 PIP joints. As such, although the pyrocarbon implant offers a potential ideal source for joint replacement, further optimization is still required for use in traumatized hands.

---

flexion, or large tendon defects that could not be repaired during the initial reconstruction, arise. Dy and colleagues[32] found the incidence of reoperation after flexor tendon surgery to be 6% in a study of 5229 patients. Of those who needed reoperation, 58% required tenolysis alone, 38% required tendon rerepair alone, and 4% required both. The initial location of the tendinous lesion is a main contributing factor to the need for secondary reconstruction. In general, flexor tendon injuries occurring in zone II have the worst prognosis. Requirements to proceed with secondary tendon procedures include complete healing of all fractures, pliable passive range of motion of the hand, adequate soft tissue coverage, and sufficient timing for maximal functional recovery after the original trauma, which takes approximately 3 months.[33,34]

Tendon adhesions The main indication to perform tenolysis is when limiting tendinous adhesions exist such that digital passive range of motion far surpasses active range of motion. Factors increasing the likelihood of adhesion formation include severe injury to the peritendinous tissues, in addition to concomitant trauma to multiple surrounding structures. The timing of tenolysis continues to be debatable. However, at least 3 months of hand therapy, whether having undergone a previous operation or not, should occur to allow for adequate tendon healing time. If the goal of near-normal digital active range of motion has not been attained by that time, tenolysis should be considered.[33]

During surgery, the patient should be actively involved in order to accurately assess the digital range of motion. In this manner, the procedure may be directed in accordance with the patient's response. The wide-awake hand surgery approach advocated by Lalonde[35] is useful. During tenolysis, release of all limiting adhesions should be performed until healthy, mobile tissue is visualized. Complete dissection of the flexor digitorum superficialis (FDS) and profundus (FDP) tendons should ideally be completed until normal tissue is reached and the tendons are freely mobilized away from each other. If dense adhesions prevent this mobilization, the FDS tendon may need to be resected. If the flexor tendons appear to be unsalvageable secondary to an abundance of scar tissue, tenolysis may be aborted and staged reconstruction may be pursued. In addition, if the critical A2 and A4 pulleys are unable to be preserved, pulley reconstruction should be considered.[33,34]

During the immediate postoperative period, management of pain and swelling should be carefully monitored in order to encourage rapid functional recovery and to decrease the chance of scar tissue formation. Range-of-motion exercises should be performed for approximately 4 to 6 weeks, taking care to perform only light activity in order to prevent injury in the early phase. Overall, an ideal posttenolysis outcome would be the ability to have a functional active range of motion using the FDS and FDP tendons.[33,34] Strickland[36] found that, in 65% of digits that underwent tenolysis, at least 50% of preoperative discrepancies between active and passive ranges of motion could be overcome. Complications that could arise as a result of tenolysis include wound breakdown, infection, and tendon rupture. In Strickland's[36] study, there was an 8% tendon rupture rate.

Tendon deficiencies Secondary tendon reconstruction should be performed in the following circumstances: the primary tendon repair failed and could not be salvaged directly; or initial tendon reconstruction was contraindicated secondary to extensive contamination, large tendon deficiency, or severe damage to peritendinous structures. In general, tendon deficiencies can be repaired using free tendon grafts via 1-stage or 2-stage tendon reconstruction. Donor tendons can be supplied by the palmaris longus, plantaris, extensor hallucis longus, extensor digitorum longus, and the FDS, if uninjured.[33] Because tendon sources are scarce at times, current research has focused on the development and clinical application of allografts (**Box 4**).

During surgery, once the sheaths and digital tunnel are properly identified and cleared of limiting scar tissue, the graft may be inserted into the flexor tendon bed within the confines of the existing pulleys. In order to optimize graft function (eg, gliding), at a minimum, the A2 and A4 pulleys should be intact, as well as part of the synovial

---

Box 4
Latest advances: tendon-bone interface allografts

As an alternative to direct tendon-to-bone suture repair of tendon injuries, reconstruction via tendon-bone interface allografts has been proposed. These composite allografts simulate a more natural, anatomic healing surface in addition to providing improved biomechanical strength.[44,45] A recent advancement in this field has been the successful physicochemical decellularization of cadaveric human, tendon-bone interface scaffolds by Bronstein and colleagues.[46] Future direction involves the clinical application of these composite allografts in humans.

---

sheath. The eventual goal is for the distal attachment of the tendon graft to be secured at the level of the distal phalanx, and for the proximal attachment to be outside no-man's land in the finger, and proximal to the zone of injury. In many instances, this requires the proximal tendon juncture to be in the distal forearm or wrist. If the injury is so extensive that it requires further soft tissue coverage, flexor sheath restoration, and/or pulley reconstruction, staged tendon reconstruction may be pursued. Instead of placing a donor tendon graft within the tendon deficiency, a Dacron-reinforced silicone implant may be used to fill the tendon defect temporarily. A flexor pseudosheath will subsequently form, allowing replacement of the implant with a donor graft during the second stage, which occurs approximately 3 months after the first-stage reconstruction.[33,34]

After surgery, the hand should be immobilized in a dorsal splint with the wrist in ~35° flexion, MCP joints in ~65° flexion, and interphalangeal joints nearing complete extension. This position prevents excessive tension from being placed on the tendon graft, in addition to encouraging vascular ingrowth. Light passive and active ranges of motion may be exercised during the first 6 weeks. Thereafter, full activity may be resumed. Overall, staged tendon reconstructions have experienced moderately good outcomes. Using LaSalle and Strickland'[37] evaluation method (total active motion [TAM] as a percentage of total passive motion), Amadio and colleagues[38] found that 54% of 117 fingers that underwent staged tendon reconstruction regained more than 50% of preoperative motion. In addition, in Wehbe and colleagues'[39] study of 155 fingers that were managed with staged flexor tendon reconstruction, the mean TAM gained after surgery from preoperative values was 74°, and the mean grip strength gained was 59% of normal. The most common complications occurring after secondary tendon reconstruction are flexion contractures, graft ruptures, and infections. The incidence rate of each of these complications, as performed in the literature review by Battiston and colleagues,[34] is 41%, 4% to 14%, and 4% to 15%, respectively.[33]

Extensor tendon injury and reconstruction
Tendon deficiencies Extensor tendon degloving injuries are more common than their flexor counterparts, given the decreased protection provided by a thin dorsal skin envelope. Multiple tendon defects from the initial hand injury or a rupture of a previously repaired extensor tendon may occur, requiring secondary operation. If direct repair is unable to be performed without excessive tension

on the repair, tendon grafting or tendon transfer may be considered.

The management of multiple extensor tendon loss is complex, and often requires careful, staged operative planning. Once stable soft tissue coverage has been achieved, silicone rods may be inserted beneath the flap. Again, fasciocutaneous flaps provide the best bed and cover for extensor tendon reconstruction. As with the implants used in staged flexor tendon reconstruction, these implants are used to form a peritendinous pseudosheath that allows later insertion of tendon grafts by promoting gliding and stability. Once the wounds have adequately healed and the patient has regained passive digital range of motion, the second stage of extensor tendon reconstruction may be performed. Fulfillment of these prerequisites is usually achieved at least 6 to 8 weeks after the initial silicone rod insertions. During the second stage, the implants are exchanged for intercalated tendon grafts.[40] The donor tendon graft is then inserted into the formed pseudosheath. The graft is either primarily attached distally to the distal, recipient tendon or directly sutured to the bone, depending on the absence or presence of active DIP joint extension, respectively. Proximally, the graft is attached proximally to the proximal, functioning motor-tendon units that remain available, ideally using a Pulvertaft weave to allow early active motion. At the end of the procedure, the DIP and PIP joints are held in full extension. Immediately after surgery, the wrist should be splinted in ~40° extension, the MCP joints in ~30° flexion, and the interphalangeal joints in total extension.[41] At 3 weeks, active digital range-of-motion exercises may be initiated, and by 8 weeks the patient may resume full digital range of activity without the use of a splint.

Although there have been limited studies regarding the role of silicone implant use in extensor tendon reconstruction, both Bevin and Hothem[42] and Adams[41] showed that use of these implants during staged extensor tendon reconstruction can restore full active extension. In 6 fingers that underwent this method of staged reconstruction, Adams[41] showed an average extension lag of 15°, and achieved greater than 90° in combined TAM of the DIP and PIP joints.[41] According to the assessment scale of Strickland and Glogovac,[43] all 6 repairs were rated fair to good in functional outcome. Some complications may arise after reconstruction, including tendinous adhesions and joint contractures, which may necessitate further reoperation such as tenolysis and capsulotomy.

Secondary Nerve Procedures

The most common indications for secondary nerve procedures include functional motor and/or sensory deficits, in addition to debilitating neuroma pain.

Motor and/or sensory deficits

Prognostic factors involved in determining the ability for nerve recovery include mechanism of injury, time from initial trauma, length of nerve defect, and complexity of associated trauma to surrounding structures. Whenever a nerve gap is present, direct end-to-end repair is always preferable. However, if the repair cannot be performed without excessive tension, nerve grafting should be considered. In general, nerve grafting to restore sensory function can be delayed, as opposed to nerve grafting to restore motor function. Time elapsed from the initial injury to the repair of motor function should be minimal, because the ability of functional return decreases with increased time elapsed from the initial injury. This inverse relationship in motor recovery is secondary to neural degeneration and scar formation, leading to permanent deficiency of target motor end plates by 1.5 years after the injury.[47] The propensity for proceeding with secondary nerve reconstruction for sensory defects increases when the injury involves critical areas of sensation.[8]

In autogenous nerve grafting, 2 donor nerves of choice are the sural nerve and the medial antebrachial cutaneous nerve.[48] Advantages of autogenous nerve grafts are that they are immunologically compatible with the patient and that they can also serve as providers of Schwann cells. A disadvantage of autogenous nerve grafts is the need for a second operative location, leading to donor-site morbidity, including sensory loss.[47]

As an alternative, both biological and synthetic nerve conduits may be used as well. However, at this time, conduits should be restricted to small-caliber sensory nerves of noncritical regions, with defects less than 3 cm in length. These nerve conduits are beneficial in that they promote axonal growth and alignment, leading to more precise, 2-point discrimination. Disadvantages of nerve conduits include their high cost, and paucity of Schwann cells. Schwann cells are essential to axonal regeneration; the need for these cells during the use of nerve conduits may be compensated for by inserting minced donor nerve into the conduit.[47,49]

Although allografts may be used, and can provide functional recovery similar to that of nerve autografts, immunosuppressive therapy for approximately 1.5 years is required, subjecting the patient to opportunistic, infectious, and neoplastic processes.[50] In order to avoid immunosuppression, nerve allografts may be decellularized, rendering them immunologically inert. However, because of this decellularization process, the same issue seen in nerve conduits arises: a lack of Schwann cells. Whitlock and colleagues[51] showed that, at 6 weeks after repair, for nerve defects less than 3 cm, the functional recovery of the treatment options discussed earlier is as follows, in order of decreasing superiority: autograft, processed allograft, and then conduit. However, their study no longer detected a difference in functional recovery by 12 weeks after reconstruction. In larger nerve defects, autografts were superior to processed allografts, and conduits were inadequate sources of repair.[47,51]

Other forms of reconstructing motor and/or sensory deficits are possible. After primary flap reconstruction, sensory deficits may still persist. Sensory recovery may be attained with a pedicle neurovascular island transfer from an adjacent finger, or a free lateral great toe pulp transfer including its neurovascular structures. If further motor reconstruction is necessary, tendon transfers should also be considered, in addition to functional free muscle transfers in complex cases.[8] In addition, nerve transfers offer a further option for restoring not only critical sensory function but motor function as well, in a timely manner. Advantages include proximity of the donor nerve to the recipient site; facilitating reinnervation; and efficient, functional restoration of a conglomerate of muscle groups with just an isolated nerve transfer (**Box 5**).[47]

Neuroma pain

Neuroma pain is a debilitating but common occurrence in the previously traumatized hand. It develops as a result of (1) impeded nerve

---

Box 5
Latest advances: Mackinnon nerve transfer
Nerve transfers may undergo the following coaptation patterns: end to end, end to side, and reverse end to side. Using these methods, Brown and Mackinnon[52] extensively described potential nerve transfers to treat residual motor and/or sensory deficits in the hand and forearm, as follows (**Fig. 5**).
Ray and Mackinnon's[53] study of 19 patients undergoing a median-to-radial nerve transfer showed promising outcomes: 95% and 63% experienced good to excellent restoration of wrist extension and finger extension, respectively, as evaluated by the Medical Research Council grading system.

---

regeneration, usually by scar formation; and (2) ectopic axonal regeneration outside the normal confinement of endoneurium at a previously repaired location. Postinjury hypersensitivity may often be confused with pain from a neuroma. In general, desensitization techniques ameliorate hypersensitivity, but not neuroma pain.[8] Treatment of the neuroma depends on 2 factors: availability of the distal nerve and sensory receptors, and critical function of the nerve involved. If the distal nerve and sensory receptors are accessible, direct nerve reconstruction or nerve grafting, after resection of the neuroma, may be performed. However, if the distal nerve and sensory receptors are not accessible, the usual treatment is resection, followed by insertion of the nerve stump into a bed of robust soft tissue. In this manner, the stump is protected from external pressure disturbance.[8] Laborde and colleagues[54] showed that dorsal translocation of neuromas results in better outcomes than simple resection with/without implantation into local muscle; the local muscle has been surmised to cause irritation secondary to contractility. Their study showed a subjective improvement in 100% of the 8 patients who underwent a dorsal translocation versus in 54% of the 13 patients who underwent a simple resection. Furthermore, the reoperation rate of each was 12.5% and 65%, respectively. In rare circumstances, the damaged nerve is of critical value, and recovery must be obtained. In this case, innervated free tissue transfer may be performed to receive the proximally regenerating nerves.[55]

Secondary Soft Tissue Procedures

Soft tissue problems requiring secondary operation include scars, web space contractures, and bulky appearance after flap reconstruction.

Web space contractures

Web space contractures, specifically of the first web space, frequently occur after trauma to the hand, and can severely limit function. These contractures can be treated by releasing the contracture and covering the resulting defect with a skin graft, local tissue rearrangement, flap coverage, or a dermal substitute (**Box 6**). The first dorsal interosseous muscle fascia is entered and partially released, followed by partial release of the adductor pollicis brevis muscle. Thumb abduction can then be obtained and secured into position using Kirschner wire fixation. Depending on surgeon preference and the size of the defect, either a split-thickness or full-thickness skin graft may be used. The skin graft may be safely secured underneath a foam or sponge dressing, which allows fluid drainage and absorption, thereby limiting fluid

Nerve Deficit	Donor Nerve → Recipient Nerve
Radial motor	Median branches to FDS → ECRB branch of radial nerve
	Median branches to FCR and PL → PIN branch of radial nerve
Radial sensory	LABC → radial sensory nerve
Median motor	AIN → median recurrent motor branch nerve
Median sensory	Ulnar-innervated 4th web space common digital nerve → median-innervated 1st web space
AIN (flexion and pronation)	ECRB branch of radial nerve → AIN
	Brachialis branch of musculocutaneous nerve → AIN
Pronator teres	ECRB branch of radial nerve → branches of pronator teres from median nerve
Ulnar motor	Distal AIN → ulnar deep motor branch
Ulnar sensory	Median sensory component of 3rd web space → ulnar sensory branch to palm

Fig. 5. Potential nerve transfers for respective nerve deficits. AIN, anterior interosseous nerve; ECRB, extensor carpi radialis brevis; FCR, flexor carpi radialis; LABC, lateral antebrachial cutaneous; PIN, posterior interosseous nerve; PL, pollicis longus. (*Adapted from* Brown JM, Mackinnon SE. Nerve transfers in the forearm and hand. Hand Clin 2008;24(4):319–40; with permission.)

accumulation beneath the graft. In this manner, stimulation of capillary ingrowth occurs, increasing the chance of graft survival. Local tissue rearrangement is another option if adjacent tissue is in favorable condition. These options include simple Z-plasties, 4-flap Z-plasties, modified double-opposing Z-plasties, jumping man flaps, and local rotational flaps.[1] Meyer and colleagues'[56] studied 103 first web space contracture revisions and concluded that simple Z-plasties were adequate in increasing skin coverage up to 1 cm, whereas double-opposing Z-plasties and local rotational flaps were successful in increasing skin coverage up to 4 cm. Furthermore, double-opposing Z-plasties were useful in creating additional depth.[56] If

---

Box 6
Latest advances: Integra

Integra is a bilayer dermal substitute, consisting of a cross-linked bovine collagen/chondroitin 6-sulfate layer and a silicone outer layer, which has recently shown promise in treating soft tissue defects of the hand. The layer applied to the wound bed encourages neovascularization, whereas the outer layer serves as protection against moisture evaporation. The outer silicone layer is removed approximately 2 to 3 weeks after placement of the dermal substitute, and is subsequently covered by a thick split-thickness skin graft. Integra has successful engraftment rates when used in wounds with exposed tendon, joint, and bone. In 2 separate literature reviews performed by Iorio and colleagues[57] and Watt and colleagues,[58] engraftment rates in complex hand wounds ranged from 87% to 100%. Although further investigations are needed to compare the outcomes of flap reconstruction with Integra, the dermal substitute already seems to serve as an excellent alternative, given its decreased donor-site morbidity and advantages in both function and aesthetic outcomes.[59]

---

free tissue transfer is necessary, fasciocutaneous flaps should be used because their malleable nature minimizes restrictive motion of the recovering thumb. An ideal and easily accessible flap for this reconstruction is the lateral arm flap (**Fig. 6**).

Bulky appearance

Functional recovery is of foremost importance after hand trauma. As such, much progress has been made toward optimal hand function after injury. In addition to improvements in function, the appearance of the hand is an important patient concern. A common complaint is the bulky appearance of the hand after undergoing fasciocutaneous flap reconstruction; the so-called biscuit phenomenon. As a result, serial debulking procedures have been performed to refine both appearance and function of the hand. These debulking operations involve staged, suction-assisted or sharp, excisional lipectomies.[60] The goal of these operations is to remove subcutaneous fat within the plane of the flap subdermis and the fascia of the hand.[61]

Major drawbacks in performing these procedures include the risk of injury to the flap's vascular pedicle, in addition to the high likelihood of needing numerous revision operations. However, 2 factors may decrease this risk: time elapsed from initial flap reconstruction and surgical approach. The surgeon should wait at least several months before separating the flap from its axial vascular pedicle, until adequate revascularization is assured. Furthermore, Reuben and colleagues[60] described the suction-assisted lipectomy approach to be safer, more effective, and to require fewer revisions compared with the sharp excisional approach. In a series of 16 flaps that underwent suction-assisted lipectomy for bulky appearance, no complications were observed, and only 12.5% of the flaps required secondary refinement for contouring enhancement.[60]

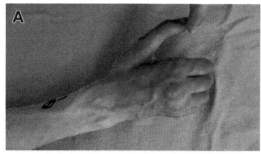

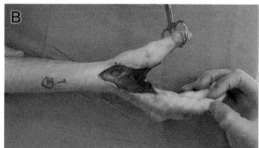

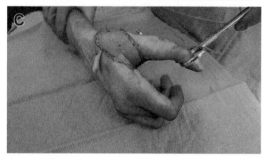

Fig. 6. (*A*) First web space contracture. (*B*) Release of the web space contracture with new tissue defect. (*C*) Reconstruction of the resultant skin defect with a lateral arm flap.

Additional flap debulking may be considered when attempting to reestablish obliterated landmarks of the hand. For example, differential refinement of subcutaneous fat may sharpen hand contour by improving topographic contrast.[58] Other procedures that may also improve appearance after flap reconstruction include complex tissue rearrangements, pulp plasties, and scar revisions.

SUMMARY

Many soft tissue defects resulting from mutilating trauma to the hand require flap coverage during initial reconstruction. The flap selection process should not only focus on matching the characteristics of the original defect but should also take into consideration the possibility of future reoperation, necessitating safe secondary flap elevation. When these factors are taken into consideration, a fasciocutaneous flap is the optimal choice for soft tissue coverage. Once initial flap reconstruction has been performed, the surgeon should wait at least several weeks for adequate revascularization and soft tissue equilibrium to occur before proceeding with flap re-elevation and subsequent operations required to regain maximal hand function. The goal is to attain optimal function and aesthetic appearance of the traumatized hand.

REFERENCES

1. Russell RC, Bueno RA, Wu TT. Secondary procedures following mutilating hand injuries. Hand Clin 2003;19:149–63.
2. Pederson WC, Lister GD. Skin flaps. In: Green DP, editor. Green's operative hand surgery. 5th edition. Philadelphia: Churchill Livingstone; 2005. p. 1648–703.
3. Kimata Y, Uchiyama K, Ebihara S, et al. Anatomic variations and technical problems of the anterolateral thigh flap: a report of 74 cases. Plast Reconstr Surg 1998;102(5):1517–23.
4. Wei FC, Jain V, Celik N, et al. Have we found an ideal soft-tissue flap? An experience with 672 anterolateral thigh flaps. Plast Reconstr Surg 2002; 109(7):2219–26.
5. Hui-Chou HG, Sulek J, Bluebond-Langner R, et al. Secondary refinements of free perforator flaps for lower extremity reconstruction. Plast Reconstr Surg 2011;127:248–57.
6. Yazar S, Lin CH, Lin YT, et al. Outcome comparison between free muscle and free fasciocutaneous flaps for reconstruction of distal third and ankle traumatic open tibial fractures. Plast Reconstr Surg 2006;117:2468–75.
7. Parrett BM, Bou-Merhi JS, Buntic RF, et al. Refining outcomes in dorsal hand coverage: consideration of aesthetics and donor-site morbidity. Plast Reconstr Surg 2010;126:1630–8.
8. Vedder NB, Hanel DP. The mangled upper extremity. In: Green DP, editor. Green's operative hand surgery. 5th edition. Philadelphia: Churchill Livingstone; 2005. p. 1587–628.
9. Rosenwasser MP, Quitkin HM. Malunion and other posttraumatic complications in the hand. In: Berger RA, editor. Hand surgery. Philadelphia: Lippincott; 2004. p. 207–15. OvidSP Web site. Available at: http://ovidsp.tx.ovid.com. Accessed September 2, 2013.
10. Buchler U, Gupta A, Ruf S. Corrective osteotomy for post-traumatic malunion of the phalanges in the hand. J Hand Surg Br 1996;21B:33–42.
11. van der Lei B, de Jonge J, Robinson PH. Correction osteotomies of phalanges and metacarpals for rotational and angular malunion: a long-term follow-up and a review of the literature. J Trauma 1993;35(6):902–8.

12. Wang H, Oswald T, Lineaweaver W. Secondary surgery following replantation. In: Weinzweig N, editor. The mutilated hand. Philadelphia: Mosby; 2005. p. 247–64.

13. Hammert WC. Hand fractures and joint injuries. In: Chang J, editor. Plastic surgery Vol. 6: hand and upper limb. Philadelphia: Saunders; 2013. p. 138–60. ExpertConsult Web site. Available at: http://www.expertconsult.com. Accessed July 16, 2013.

14. Barton NJ. Fractures of the shafts of the phalanges of the hand. Hand 1979;11:119–33.

15. Borgeskov S. Conservative therapy for fractures of the phalanges and metacarpals. Acta Chir Scand 1967;133:123–30.

16. Stern PJ. Fractures of the metacarpals and phalanges. In: Green DP, editor. Green's operative hand surgery. 5th edition. Philadelphia: Churchill Livingstone; 2005. p. 277–341.

17. Baumeister S, Germann GK. Principles of internal fixation. In: Weinzweig N, editor. The mutilated hand. Philadelphia: Mosby; 2005. p. 405.

18. Baumeister S, Germann GK. Principles of bony reconstruction. In: Weinzweig N, editor. The mutilated hand. Philadelphia: Mosby; 2005. p. 391–3.

19. Bishop AT. Vascularized bone grafting. In: Green DP, editor. Green's operative hand surgery. 5th edition. Philadelphia: Churchill Livingstone; 2005. p. 1777–808.

20. Jupiter JB, Koniuch MP, Smith RJ. The management of delayed union and nonunion of the metacarpals and phalanges. J Hand Surg 1985; 10A(4):457–66.

21. Rogers SN, Lakshmiah SR, Narayan B, et al. A comparison of the long-term morbidity following deep circumflex iliac and fibula free flaps for reconstruction following head and neck cancer. Plast Reconstr Surg 2003;112(6):1517–25.

22. Choudry UH, Bakri K, Moran SL, et al. The vascularized medial femoral condyle periosteal bone flap for the treatment of recalcitrant bony nonunions. Ann Plast Surg 2008;60:174–80.

23. Shin AY, Amadio PC. Stiff finger joints. In: Green DP, editor. Green's operative hand surgery. 5th edition. Philadelphia: Churchill Livingstone; 2005. p. 417–60.

24. Young VL, Wray RC, Weeks PM. The surgical management of stiff joints in the hand. Plast Reconstr Surg 1978;62(6):835–41.

25. Ellis PR, Tsai TM. Management of the traumatized joint of the finger. Clin Plast Surg 1989;16(3):457–73.

26. Stern PJ, Fulton DB. Distal interphalangeal joint arthrodesis: an analysis of complications. J Hand Surg Am 1992;17A:1139–45.

27. Leibovic SJ, Strickland JW. Arthrodesis of the proximal interphalangeal joint of the finger: comparison of the use of the Herbert screw with other fixation methods. J Hand Surg Am 1994;19A(2):181–8.

28. Cook SD, Beckenbaugh RD, Redondo J, et al. Long-term follow-up of pyrolytic carbon metacarpophalangeal implants. J Bone Joint Surg Am 1999;81(5):635–48.

29. McGuire DT, White CD, Carter SL, et al. Pyrocarbon proximal interphalangeal joint arthroplasty: outcomes of a cohort study. J Hand Surg Eur Vol 2012;37:490–6.

30. Ono S, Shauver MJ, Chang KW, et al. Outcomes of pyrolitic carbon arthroplasty for the proximal interphalangeal joint at 44 months mean follow-up. Plast Reconstr Surg 2012;129(5):1139–50.

31. Chan K, Ayeni O, McKnight L, et al. Pyrocarbon versus silicone proximal interphalangeal joint arthroplasty: a systematic review. Plast Reconstr Surg 2013;131:114–24.

32. Dy CJ, Daluiski A, Do HT, et al. The epidemiology of reoperation after flexor tendon repair. J Hand Surg 2012;37A:919–24.

33. Tang JB. Flexor tendon injury and reconstruction. In: Chang J, editor. Plastic surgery Vol. 6: hand and upper limb. Philadelphia: Saunders; 2013. p. 178–209. ExpertConsult Web site. Available at: http://www.expertconsult.com. Accessed July 16, 2013.

34. Battiston B, Triolo PF, Bernardi A, et al. Secondary repair of flexor tendon injuries. Injury 2013;44: 340–5.

35. Lalonde DH. Reconstruction of the hand with wide awake surgery. Clin Plast Surg 2011;38(4): 761–9.

36. Strickland JW. Flexor tendon surgery: part 2: free tendon grafts and tenolysis. J Hand Surg Br 1989;14:368–82.

37. LaSalle WB, Strickland JW. An evaluation of the two-stage flexor tendon reconstruction technique. J Hand Surg 1983;8:263–7.

38. Amadio PC, Wood MB, Cooney WP, et al. Staged flexor tendon reconstruction in the fingers and hand. J Hand Surg 1988;13A:559–62.

39. Wehbe MA, Hunter JM, Schneider LH, et al. Two-stage flexor-tendon reconstruction. J Bone Joint Surg Am 1986;68(5):752–63.

40. Gonzalez MH, Weinzweig N, Graf CN, et al. Management of the ulnar mutilating injury. In: Weinzweig N, editor. The mutilated hand. Philadelphia: Mosby; 2005. p. 87–95.

41. Adams BD. Staged extensor tendon reconstruction in the finger. J Hand Surg Am 1997;22A:833–7.

42. Bevin AG, Hothem AL. The use of silicone rods under split-thickness skin grafts for reconstruction of extensor tendon injuries. Hand 1978; 10(3):254–8.

43. Strickland JW, Glogovac SV. Digital function following flexor tendon repair in zone II: a comparison of immobilization and controlled passive motion techniques. J Hand Surg 1980;5:537–43.

44. Zhang W, Pan W, Zhang M, et al. In vivo evaluation of two types of bioactive scaffold used for tendon-bone interface healing in the reconstruction of anterior cruciate ligament. Biotechnol Lett 2011;33:837–44.

45. Rodeo SA, Arnoczky SP, Torzilli PA, et al. Tendon-healing in a bone tunnel: a biomechanical and histological study in the dog. J Bone Joint Surg Am 1993;75:1795–803.

46. Bronstein JA, Woon CY, Farnebo S, et al. Physicochemical decellularization of composite flexor tendon-bone interface grafts. Plast Reconstr Surg 2013;132:94–102.

47. Boyd KU, Nimigan AS, Mackinnon SE. Nerve reconstruction in the hand and upper extremity. Clin Plast Surg 2011;38:643–60.

48. Birch R. Nerve repair. In: Green DP, editor. Green's operative hand surgery. 5th edition. Philadelphia: Churchill Livingstone; 2005. p. 1075–112.

49. Agnew SP, Dumanian GA. Technical use of synthetic conduits for nerve repair. J Hand Surg Am 2010;35(5):838–41.

50. Mackinnon SE, Doolabh VB, Novak CB, et al. Clinical outcome following nerve allograft transplantation. Plast Reconstr Surg 2001;107(6):1419–29.

51. Whitlock EL, Tuffaha SH, Luciano JP, et al. Processed allografts and type I collagen conduits for repair of peripheral nerve gaps. Muscle Nerve 2009;39(6):787–99.

52. Brown JM, Mackinnon SE. Nerve transfers in the forearm and hand. Hand Clin 2008;24(4):319–40.

53. Ray WZ, Mackinnon SE. Clinical outcomes following median to radial nerve transfers. J Hand Surg Am 2011;36(2):201–8.

54. Laborde KJ, Kalisman M, Tsai TM. Results of surgical treatment of painful neuromas of the hand. J Hand Surg 1982;7(2):190–3.

55. Wiesman IM, Mackinnon SE. Painful digits and amputation stumps of the hand. In: Weinzweig N, editor. The mutilated hand. Philadelphia: Mosby; 2005. p. 533–46.

56. Meyer RD, Gould JS, Nicholson B. Revision of the first web space: technics and results. South Med J 1981;74(10):1204–8.

57. Iorio ML, Shuck J, Attinger CE. Wound healing in the upper and lower extremities: a systematic review on the use of acellular dermal matrices. Plast Reconstr Surg 2012;130(Suppl 2):232S–41S.

58. Watt AJ, Friedrich JB, Huang JI. Advances in treating skin defects of the hand: skin substitutes and negative-pressure wound therapy. Hand Clin 2012;28:519–28.

59. Stiefel D, Schiestl C, Meuli M. Integra artificial skin for burn scar revision in adolescents and children. Burns 2010;36(1):114–20.

60. Reuben CM, Bastidas N, Sharma S. Power-assisted suction lipectomy of fasciocutaneous flaps in the extremities. Ann Plast Surg 2010;65(1):60–5.

61. Higgins JP, Seruya M. Visual subunits of the hand: proposed guidelines for revision surgery after flap reconstruction of the traumatized hand. J Reconstr Microsurg 2011;27:551–8.

Optimizing Functional and Aesthetic Outcomes of Upper Limb Soft Tissue Reconstruction

Cenk Cayci, MD[a], Brian T. Carlsen, MD[b],
Michel Saint-Cyr, MD[b],*

KEYWORDS

- Functional outcomes • Aesthetic outcomes • Upper limb • Soft tissue • Reconstruction

KEY POINTS

- Optimal functional and aesthetic outcomes for hand reconstruction depend on optimizing the ideal flap for any given defect.
- Having a wider range of flap options in the armamentarium provides more flexibility in achieving these goals.
- The hand and reconstructive surgeon has to consider multiple factors before surgery and flap selection: patient body habitus, flap donor site options, and characteristics relative to the recipient site defect.
- Anatomic and functional variations should be taken into consideration in selecting the type of reconstruction.
- Local flaps provide reconstruction of the defects with like tissues and prevent additional morbidity to the other areas of the body.
- Adjuncts like primary donor site closure, suprafascial flap harvest, use of full-thickness skin grafting, and local rotation flaps can all improve the donor site closure and cosmesis.
- Free tissue transfer provides a wide variety of options for upper extremity reconstruction.
- Having a greater availability of flap choices allows surgeons to be more selective in choosing the optimal fasciocutaneous flap donor site.
- Targeted debulking, redefining topographic regions by designing asymmetric skin excisions, and recreating natural crease lines that border adjacent aesthetic units may improve the aesthetic outcome.
- Measures such as peripheral flap thinning, recipient skin edge elevation and resection to healthy nonscarred tissue, and meticulous inset for muscle flaps with proper overlap and native skin marsupialization may all improve the aesthetic outcomes after upper extremity reconstruction.

INTRODUCTION

Posttraumatic hand deformities represent a unique challenge for hand and reconstructive surgeons. Goals of treatment should include not only restoration of function but also restoration of preinjury aesthetics. The hand and upper extremity play an important role socially and form the fundamental basis of communication and self-expression. Although restoring hand function remains a

Conflicts of Interest: None.
[a] Division of Plastic and Reconstructive Surgery, College of Medicine, Mayo Clinic, 200 First Street Southwest, Rochester, MN 55905, USA; [b] Division of Plastic and Reconstructive Surgery, College of Medicine, Mayo Clinic, 200 First Street Southwest, Rochester, MN 55905, USA
* Corresponding author.
E-mail address: saintcyr.michel@mayo.edu

Hand Clin 30 (2014) 225–238
http://dx.doi.org/10.1016/j.hcl.2014.01.005

hand.theclinics.com

principal consideration, special attention needs to be placed on the final reconstructed hand appearance. We have long moved past the goal of only achieving wound closure and restoring function. Success in hand reconstruction is now measured by reestablishing preinjury function and, just as importantly, preinjury aesthetic appearance. Careful flap donor site selection and flap inset both play a critical role in achieving these goals.

Hand, wrist, and distal forearm injuries are common and frequently present with exposed bone, tendons, muscle, and nerves. The immediate priority is adequate debridement of the devitalized tissue, fracture fixation to create a stable reconstructive platform, and repair of tendon and all critical neurovascular structures. Once these goals have been achieved, attention can be concentrated on optimizing soft tissue coverage.[1–12] Various options exist for soft tissue closure, including local, regional, and distant pedicle flaps as well as free flaps.[13–19] Because of the distinct contour characteristics and relative paucity of subcutaneous tissue in the hand, posttraumatic flap reconstructions may require secondary debulking to improve contour. Optimal flap selection is determined by replacing like with like and minimizing donor site morbidity. A beautiful reconstruction resulting in a poor or disfiguring donor site is a neutral outcome and trade-off and should be avoided. Careful selection of flap type and donor site, as well as meticulous flap insetting and aesthetic unit–directed preparation of the recipient site yield better results.[20,21] In this article, the aspects of optimal flap selection, inset, recipient site preparation, and secondary revisions to maximize aesthetic outcome are discussed.

Before any flap-based soft tissue coverage, proper wound debridement remains fundamental (**Fig. 1**). Low infection rates are reported after hand trauma, even in cases of significant contamination or bone or hardware exposure. In a series reported by Parrett and colleagues[22] with total 125 free flaps in 124 patients, reported infection rate was 4.8%, with a mean follow-up of 18 months. These investigators attributed this relatively low infection rate to aggressive debridement and rapid flap coverage. All patients underwent initial debridement within the first 24 hours of the trauma, with repeated debridement as indicated (mean of 1.6 per patient). The flap coverage was performed with a mean time of 5.6 days from the time of injury.[22]

PATIENT BODY HABITUS

Flap selection should take into consideration patient body habitus, body mass index (BMI), and available donor sites. Donor site characteristics such as skin color, dermal and subcutaneous tissue thickness, glabrous versus nonglabrous skin, and associated flap pedicle length all play a determining role. Ideally, skin defects should be replaced with like-skin flaps, which have the advantage of being reelevated for secondary surgeries. Patients with a high BMI are often better served with muscle flaps or fascial flaps. Muscle flaps atrophy and contour accordingly, whereas large and thick fasciocutaneous flaps may require significant debulking. Adipose tissue distribution in the body also varies, for example, patients with an unsuitable and thick anterolateral thigh (ALT) donor site may have an excellent scapular or thoracodorsal artery perforator (TDAP) flap donor site. In patients with a high BMI, flaps such as groin or superficial circumflex iliac artery perforator, sural artery perforator, TDAP, and scapular as well as adipofascial flaps may be excellent alternatives because of their relative thinness (**Fig. 2**).

ANATOMIC LOCATION

The type of reconstruction for the upper extremity is highly dependent on the anatomic location of the

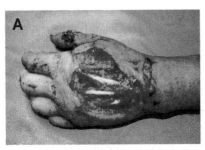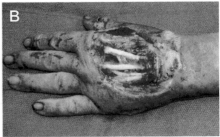

Fig. 1. (*A*) Dorsal degloving left hand injury before surgical debridement. (*B*) Dorsal degloving injury after aggressive wound debridement. Debridement was started just outside the zone of injury to enter a natural untraumatized tissue plane, similar to extirpating a tumor. An upper extremity tourniquet was used during the debridement to minimize bleeding and facilitate debridement. Note that the smaller proximal wound found in (*A*) was combined with the larger one to create a single uniform wound aesthetic unit.

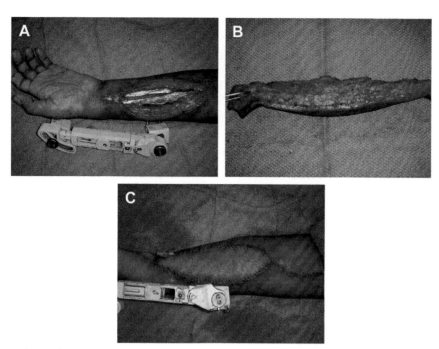

Fig. 2. (A) Distal volar forearm soft tissue loss with exposed flexor tendons and external fixator for stabilization of distal radius fracture. (B) The recipient site skin and subcutaneous tissue thickness was measured and matched with a similarly sized parascapular flap donor site. A pinch test was used and divided by half to assess the flap donor site thickness and compare it with the recipient wound thickness. (C) Stable coverage of the forearm wound with a parascapular flap. Note that the peripheral scar of the original wound bed was debrided for better cosmesis. The longitudinal scar was also excised to create a more aesthetically uniform reconstruction.

defect. There are significant anatomic and functional variations on the upper extremity. For example, glabrous thick skin, which would potentially resist the shear forces, is the major requirement for reconstruction of the volar aspect of the hand and fingers, whereas a thinner nonglabrous reconstruction is necessary for the dorsal surface of the hand.

Dorsal Hand Wound

The goals of reconstruction in this area are to provide thin and pliable soft tissue coverage, which allows proper tendon gliding, bony healing, and early rehabilitation. The coverage options for this area include reverse radial forearm, with possible adipofascial, fasciocutaneous, or fascial modifications, posterior interosseous flap, groin flap, Integra (Lifecell Corporation in Branchburg, NJ, USA)/skin graft, or free flap reconstruction. If there are exposed tendons without intact paratenon, consideration of coverage that delivers a gliding surface for the tendons is crucial. If a reverse radial forearm fasciocutaneous flap reconstruction is the choice of reconstruction, a suprafascial harvest can help minimize donor site morbidity and provide a thinner flap, with potentially less of a pincushioning effect in

the recipient site. Other modifications include the radial forearm flap with fascia only, or as a pedicle perforator flap with skin harvested subfascially or suprafascially (**Fig. 3**), or with fascia alone. These modifications also help to maximize donor site aesthetic outcomes.

Thumb Pulp Defect

A thumb pulp defect is a highly specialized area that consists of sensate glabrous skin, which is exposed to shear forces. Goals of reconstruction should include restoration of sensation with a flap that is resistant to shear forces to allow for adequate pinch. Options include cross-finger flap (CFF), Moberg flap, heterodigital island flap, first dorsal metacarpal artery (FDMA) flap, sensate first web space flap (first dorsal metatarsal artery flap), and free sensate toe pulp flap. The Moberg flap is an excellent option, in that it restores immediate 2-point discrimination with identical glabrous skin. Limitations of the Moberg flap may include donor site skin grafting, which can be avoided with local triangular transposition flaps for primary donor site closure (**Fig. 4**). Extension splinting is also important postoperatively to avoid interphalangeal joint (IPJ) contracture.[23] An FDMA flap is

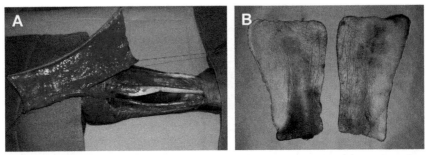

Fig. 3. (*A*) Suprafascial harvest of a radial forearm flap (RFF), with preservation of fascia over the volar muscle bellies and flexor tendons. (*B*) Anterior-posterior view of 2 RFFs after injection with methylene blue to assess vascular territories. The suprafascially harvested RFF on the right and subfascially harvested RFF on the left show similar vascular territories.

a good local option, which uses expendable tissue from the dorsal aspect of the index, with minimal donor site morbidity. The FDMA flap comprises nonglabrous skin, with variable sensibility and 2-point discrimination.[24] A more technically challenging option is the free toe pulp flap, which can provide sensate, glabrous tissue for the thumb pulp. In addition, there is no further compromise of hand function, because the flap is harvested remotely, using like tissue, with highly acceptable end results.[25]

First Web Space Defect

The goals of reconstruction for this area are to provide skin and soft tissue coverage with enough bulk to fill the complex three-dimensional defect created by contracture release. The aesthetic aspect of the web space must be recreated with a flap that contours this area nicely and obliterates dead space appropriately yet is not too bulky or thin. A bulky flap limits key pinch, and an overly thin flap may not fill the substantial dead space created after aggressive contracture release. The optimal flap should also act as a buttress to keep the first web space open and prevent further adduction contracture. Options for reconstruction include the reverse radial forearm, the posterior interosseous flap, the groin flap, the FDMA flap, and fasciocutaneous free flaps such as the lateral arm and ALT or TDAP flaps. The posterior interosseous

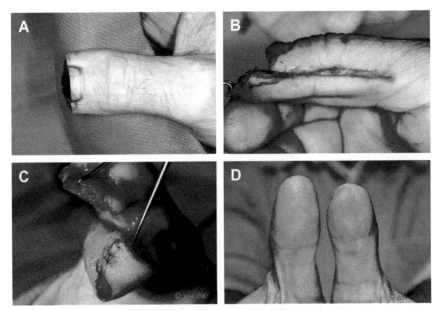

Fig. 4. (*A*) Left thumb middistal phalangeal level amputation. (*B*) Moberg flap elevation and advancement. The interphalangeal joint is flexed accordingly to maximize advancement and minimize closing tension. Additional advancement can be achieved by converting the Moberg flap to an island flap. (*C*) Cupping of the distal portion of the Moberg flap for better contouring, note the excision of small triangle distally. (*D*) Outcome.

artery flap is a traditional regional flap for the first web space. It is most commonly used as a reversed pedicled flap but can also be harvested as a free flap.[26] The advantages of the flap are its harvest from the same affected side and preservation of the main arterial inflow to the hand. The dorsal forearm skin and the first web space have a good color/texture match. One disadvantage of the flap is that it is a technically demanding flap, with variable anatomy.[27] The lateral arm flap, which can be raised as a sensate flap by including the posterior brachial cutaneous nerve, provides a good option for first web space reconstruction.[28,29] The advantages of this flap are numerous and include the provision of a good color/texture match, flap harvesting from the same extremity, limited donor site morbidity with possible primary closure, and disguising the incision within clothing. This flap on cross section is trapezoidal, and therefore fills the first web space three-dimensional defect well. Alternatively, muscle flaps in combination with sheet split-thickness skin graft (STSG) rather then meshed grafting can also be used for reconstruction of the first web space and have the advantage of excellent dead space obliteration and acceptable appearance. Unlike fasciocutaneous flaps, muscle flaps atrophy and mold themselves to the recipient site with minimal bulk and rarely need revision (**Fig. 5**).

Volar Finger Defect

The goals of reconstruction in this area are to provide durable, sensate soft tissue coverage, with resistance to shear forces. Options are healing by secondary intention, revision amputation, thenar flap, homodigital island flaps, V-Y advancement flaps, CFF, reverse homodigital island flap, and so forth (**Fig. 6**). An established method to reconstruct this area is the CFF.[30] The technique uses local, relatively expandable tissue for reconstruction, with minimal donor site morbidity.[31] Flap can be harvested as skin (conventional CFF), soft tissue only (reverse CFF), or as an innervated flap.[32] This is a reliable and technically easy option but requires initial immobilization of the fingers, which may result in joint stiffness, 2 stages to complete the reconstruction, and provide a nonglabrous tissue for an area that is under shear forces. To increase flap volume to best recreate the pulp, an extended CFF can be harvested with additional dorsal subcutaneous tissue. This strategy provides better pulp volume and padding and, in turn, produces a less atrophied and skeletonized fingertip pulp, as seen with a conventional CFF (**Fig. 7**). We prefer to cover the donor site with a full-thickness rather than STSG for improved

appearance. We also convert partial donor defects into a complete aesthetic unit from the distal IPJ (DIPJ) to the proximal IPJ (PIPJ) and bilateral mid-axial lines to place wound borders along natural creases for less conspicuous scarring (**Fig. 8**). Many homodigital anterograde island flaps have been described and, like the Moberg flap for the thumb, can offer excellent soft tissue coverage for digital tip defects.[33–37] These flaps have the benefit of providing instant 2-point discrimination, excellent color and texture match, with equivalent adjacent glabrous sensate skin (**Fig. 9**). A technically more challenging technique is the reverse homodigital island flap.[38,39] This flap is elevated from the lateral aspect of the proximal phalanx, with an arterial pedicle centered in the flap. The retrograde blood supply flow came from the abundant vascular network between the radial and ulnar digital artery. This 1-stage procedure, without the requirement of a period of immobilization or injury to other fingers, can provide a wide rotational arc and larger flap size and is an excellent procedure for distal digital soft tissue defects. The disadvantages include the sacrifice of 1 of 2 proper digital arteries and additional damage to an injured finger.

FLAP SELECTION

The literature is replete with various flap options for hand coverage, including muscle, fasciocutaneous, fascial, and venous flaps.[13–19,40,41] In earlier studies, success was often equated with flap survival.[15,42–46] Flap failure rates remain relatively low.[22] The unique functional and aesthetic properties of the upper extremity require that outcomes are measured by restoring normal or near-normal preinjury function and appearance. Every patient has a unique set of flap donor site options and recipient defect characteristics, which are mutually inclusive. Important factors to consider include skin type, skin color, flap thickness relative to the recipient site, and future need for secondary surgeries (eg, bone grafting, nerve and tendon grafting, debulking). Bulky fasciocutaneous flaps, which are unsightly and limit function, should be avoided in favor of fascial flaps or muscle flaps, which atrophy for better contouring.

Fasciocutaneous Flaps

Fasciocutaneous flaps remain an excellent means of restoring preinjury appearance and sensation in the upper extremity. Their simple harvest combined with ease of defatting and reelevation for secondary surgeries make them an obvious choice. Experience with numerous pedicle fasciocutaneous flaps (eg, groin, CFF, thenar, and thoracoabdominal flaps) has shown that they can be

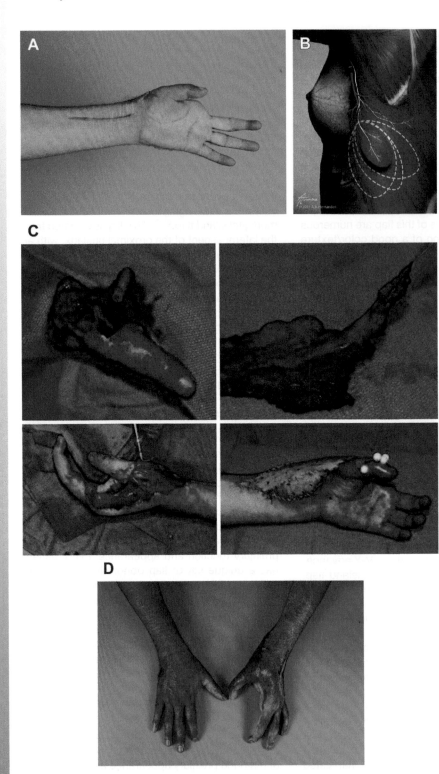

Fig. 5. (A) Left hand crush injury, with resulting first web space adduction contracture, and nonunion of first metacarpal. (B) The free muscle-sparing latissimus dorsal (MSLD) flap, based on the descending branch of the thoracodorsal artery (TDA). (C) Sequence of surgery showing use of a vascularized pedicled second metacarpal flap for nonunion correction of the base of the first metacarpal, second ray amputation and web space coverage with a free MSLD flap based on the descending branch of the TDA. Note that to avoid additional donor site morbidity, the overlying skin paddle from the MSLD flap was used as an STSG source. This principle can be applied to all muscle flap harvests to improve donor site cosmesis. (D) Postoperative view 6 weeks after surgery, with improved first web space and minimal muscle flap bulk.

safely divided from their axial vascular pedicle weeks to months after insetting (**Fig. 10**). This factor highlights the important contribution of neovascularization within the peripheral flap edge and, to some degree, the underlying recipient bed.[47–51] Flaps inset into poorly vascularized recipient tissue may require longer healing before division of their pedicle. The principle of peripheral vascular

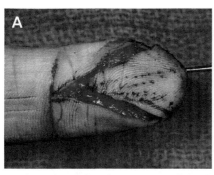 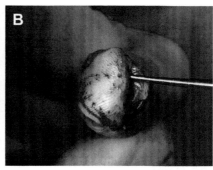

Fig. 6. (*A*) V-Y advancement flap for coverage of distal tip defect. To maximize cosmesis of the tip, the flap base should equal the width of the nail plate and not the entire stump width. This strategy avoids creating a chopstick deformity of the distal tip, which is unsightly, especially in women. (*B*) The volar V-Y flap is advanced 10% more then required, above the nail bed to avoid a hook nail deformity from secondary contracture.

ingrowth also allows for aggressive defatting of fasciocutaneous free flaps 3 to 6 months after initial surgery. We prefer to aggressively defat fasciocutaneous flaps with lipoaspiration alone and wait for secondary postlipoaspiration skin contracture before excising any redundant tissue, which allows for maximal blood supply preservation and is safe (**Fig. 11**). Care must be taken to not perform overzealous lipoaspiration in combination with direct skin excision for risks for partial flap failure. If both procedures are combined (lipoaspiration and direct skin excision), less than 50% of the flap periphery should be incised to maintain adequate blood supply. In addition, for patients requiring secondary surgeries, debulking can also be performed at this time. Removal of excess subcutaneous fat and the resultant skin redundancy often allow for a more favorable reorientation and excision of scars.

The concept by Higgins and Seruya,[52] proposed thenar, hypothenar, midpalm, distal palm, dorsal hand, volar forearm, and dorsal forearm subunits as "visual subunits of the hand" in an effort to guide restoration of the natural hand. These

investigators' proposed guidelines for debulking surgery included flap skin encompassing a single subunit, leaving the scars along the margins of the subunit, differential thinning of the subcutaneous fat between areas of contrast, and purposeful designing of unequal skin closure lines to create differences in soft tissue projection and as well as natural skin creases.

In a series by Parrett and colleagues,[22] 88% of ALT flaps required future debulking, with a mean of 2 debulking procedures per flap. This finding was despite initial thinning of most of the ALT flaps before inset. Flaps that may provide less bulk then the ALT flap include the lateral arm and radial forearm free flaps. Nevertheless, even these flaps have thick subcutaneous components in many patients.[40,41,53] Parrett and colleagues[22] reported 62% rate of debulking for radial forearm free flaps (**Fig. 12**). There are also donor site disadvantages with fasciocutaneous flaps, including a greater need for skin grafting of the donor site and higher breakdown rates.[22] This increased breakdown is likely caused by attempts for primary closure under tension or skin grafting over

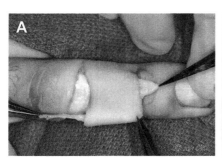 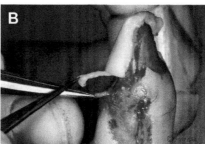

Fig. 7. (*A*) Extended CFF with additional subcutaneous tissue harvested distally to increase flap volume for better pulp padding and contouring. Note that a dorsal digital sensory branch was also incorporated into the flap to anastomose to the recipient digital nerve. (*B*) Neurorraphy between the dorsal sensory branch incorporated within the CFF and recipient ulnar digital nerve.

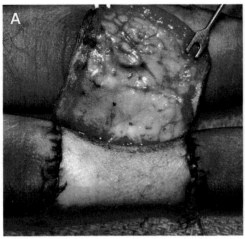
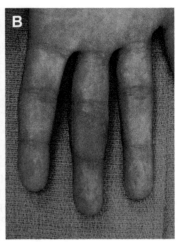

Fig. 8. (*A*) Images showing elevated CFF from dorsal middle phalanx of the right ring finger. Flap incision lines are kept with natural creases to help minimize final scarring. A thin full-thickness skin graft is preferred over an STSG to improve cosmesis and minimize contracture. Note that the skin graft is placed before flap inset to facilitate coverage. Flap donor site is converted to an aesthetic unit from the PIPJ to the DIPJ and midaxial lines. (*B*) Well-healed CFF after division and inset at 8 weeks.

tendons in the radial forearm free flap donor site (**Fig. 13**).

Several techniques have been described to thin the ALT flap, including the adipocutaneous flap, the adipofascial flap, and delayed debulking. Agostini and colleagues[54] reported the systematic review of the ALT flap adipofascial configuration. Even with adipofascial modification, a delayed debulking rate was reported in 32% (51/163 flaps) of cases.

Another proposed method for debulking fasciocutaneous free flaps is to excise the skin and use it as a full-thickness skin graft. Lin and colleagues[55] reported their series of 12 free ALT flap revisions. The epidermis and most of the dermis were harvested from the flap, regrafted on the defatted

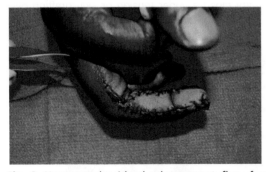

Fig. 9. Neurovascular island advancement flap, for coverage of a distal tip defect of the right middle finger. Note the significant advancement (1 cm) that can be achieved with this flap. This flap offers instant 2-point discrimination and represents well the functional and aesthetic goals of replacing like with like.

wound, and fixed with tie-over dressing for 7 days. Except for 2 cases with small areas of superficial skin loss, all grafted skin survived. The average thickness of the removed fat was 8.3 ± 2.6 mm. These investigators recommended a single-stage debulking procedure of the hand after free flap reconstruction, contrary to conventional techniques, which usually cannot provide 1-stage adequate debulking.

Muscle Flaps

Muscle flaps covered with STSG can provide good or excellent appearance, contour, and color match, with less required debulking.[22] This situation is likely caused by atrophy of the muscle, which results in a good contour match. Also, well-perfused muscle flaps can facilitate STSG take, resulting in an excellent color match with the recipient site.[56] Sheet STSGs have a better aesthetic appearance compared with meshed STSG.[22] Better understanding of the flap anatomy has also provided the use of partial muscle flaps (eg, muscle sparing: latissimus dorsi, vastus lateralis, rectus abdominis flaps) for web space, dorsal hand, and wrist coverage, in which the flap size harvested is tailored to the defect size to avoid unnecessary bulk. This technique allows for custom-designed flaps, with preservation of donor muscle function and minimal morbidity.[42,43] The partial superior latissimus flap selectively harvests the superior portion of the latissimus, which is very thin. The free descending branch muscle-sparing latissimus dorsi flap is a viable alternative, which has the advantage of providing an easy and simple

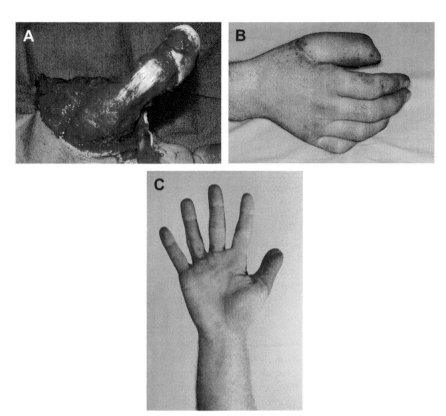

Fig. 10. (*A*) Right thumb avulsion injury, with significant circumferential soft tissue loss. (*B*) Three-month postoperative appearance, after reconstruction with a pedicle groin flap. (*C*) Postoperative result 6 months later, after direct elliptical excision of redundant skin and lipoaspiration.

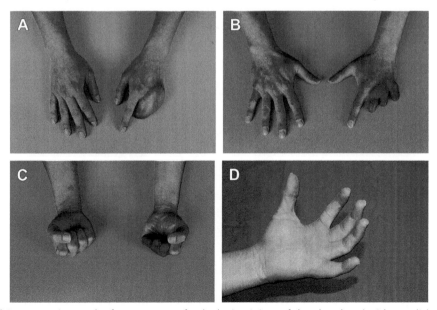

Fig. 11. (*A*) Postoperative result after coverage of a degloving injury of the ulnar hand with a pedicle groin flap. (*B*) Result 9 months postoperatively after serial lipoaspiration and direct excision. (*C*) Final range of motion with metacarpophalangeal joint flexion at 9 months. (*D*) Flap syndactyly correction allows for individualization of the digits and use of a customized prosthesis for improved cosmesis.

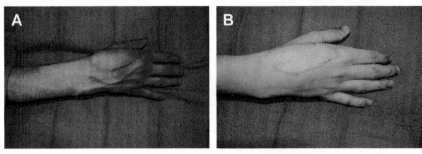

Fig. 12. (*A*) Pedicle radial forearm flap 6 months postoperatively with residual bulk and slight pincushioning effect. (*B*) Radial forearm flap after lipoaspiration 10 mL, with improved contour.

dissection because of its proximity to the anterior border of the muscle (see **Fig. 5**B).[57–59] The partial medial rectus flap can be tangentially thinned on its superficial surface before inset. Lower rates for revisions are reported in partial muscle flaps versus nonpartial muscle flaps.[22]

Fascial Flaps

Fascial flaps (ALT fascia, lateral arm fascia, dorsal thoracic fascia, and temporoparietal fascia) with STSG are very thin and pliable and, thus, match dorsal hand skin well.[14,18,19,41,44] Donor site

morbidity is minimal, because no muscle is harvested, and the donor site is closed primarily without skin grafting. Wounds of multiple sizes can be covered: the temporoparietal fascia and lateral arm fascia flaps are preferred for smaller defects and the ALT fascia and dorsal thoracic fascia flaps for larger defects.[14,19,44] Unless a thin fasciocutaneous flap can be used, fascial flaps are an excellent alternative for moderate-sized to large dorsal hand wounds, allowing a single-staged procedure, with minimal need for revision surgery. In the presence of exposed hardware or need for future reconstructive procedures,

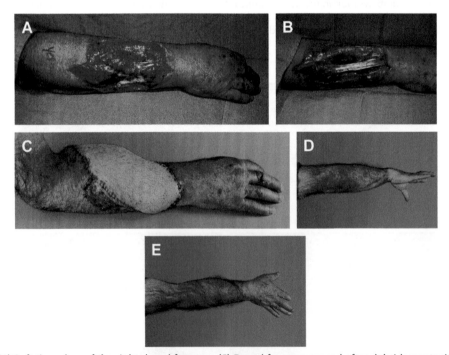

Fig. 13. (*A*) Soft tissue loss of the right dorsal forearm. (*B*) Dorsal forearm wound after debridement with conversion to a clean wound. Note that the defect was increased slightly to achieve well-vascularized nontraumatized wound edges for better flap inset and final cosmesis. (*C*) Four weeks postoperative result after coverage with a free ALT flap. Note overall bulkiness of the flap and need for an STSG. (*D*) Lateral view 12 months postoperatively after serial lipoaspiration and direct excision of ALT and STSG. (*E*) Posterior-anterior view at 12 months postoperatively, with decreased bulk and improved cosmesis.

a thicker flap, such as muscle or fasciocutaneous, may be warranted.[22]

Venous Flaps

Arterialized venous free flaps represent a reliable and safe option for resurfacing hand and finger defects.[60] Easy and fast harvesting because of the visible venous vascular system is an advantage. These flaps are thin and pliable and can be easily adjusted to the needs of the defect without sacrificing a major artery at the donor site. They can be transferred not only as a pure skin flap without fascia but as a composite flap, including tendons, nerves, and additional veins for grafting purposes. All of these advantages make it an optimal choice for reconstruction of small to moderate hand and digital defects when conventional flaps are unavailable. Arterialized venous flaps are often harvested from the volar forearm in the suprafascial plane, allowing them to be very thin and pliable, matching the surrounding dorsal hand and digital skin, with minimal donor site morbidity. Arterialized venous flaps provide coverage but can also be used as flow-through bypass for digital revascularization.[60] Additional subcutaneous efferent veins are used to establish venous drainage. The major limiting factor for arterialized free venous flaps is the defect size. Published series have shown good results using venous flaps for hand reconstruction; they should be considered as a first-line choice for small to moderate-sized defects when possible.[61–63]

Parrett and colleagues[22] conducted a study to determine the aesthetic appearance and need for revision surgery of flaps after dorsal hand coverage. These investigators compared 4 different flap groups (muscle with skin graft, fasciocutaneous, fascia with skin graft, and 2 venous flaps). Aesthetic outcomes were blindly graded by cosmetic-focused plastic surgeons and nonphysician aestheticians. Venous flaps scored the highest mean value, and the fasciocutaneous flaps scored the lowest mean ratio for overall aesthetic appearance, with muscle and fascia flaps scoring significantly better than the fasciocutaneous flaps. In terms of need for future debulking, venous flaps required no debulking (0%) and fascial flaps required less debulking than muscle flaps (5.8% vs 32%). Most fasciocutaneous flaps required debulking (67%). Partial muscle flaps required less debulking when compared with traditional muscle flaps (7% vs 37%).[22]

FLAP INSETTING

Proper attention to detail during flap insetting is crucial for maximizing aesthetic outcomes. Fasciocutaneous flaps should be harvested slightly larger than the defect to avoid peripheral tension caused by flap-recipient site discrepancies in thickness. Pincushioning effect can be limited by peripheral thinning of the flap and adequate undermining and elevation of the recipient wound skin edges to smoothen insetting transition. Also, any scarring from the defect skin edges should be excised up to healthy tissue to avoid any further secondary wound contracture and pincushioning effect. This excision should be made before final flap harvest and skin paddle incision, so as to not underestimate final flap size. This strategy also facilitates and creates a more natural and gradual flap-recipient bed transition (**Fig. 14**). Choice of proper donor site is also key to avoid flap-recipient site mismatches with regards to thickness. Reverse fasciocutaneous flaps tend to undergo more bulkiness and pincushioning effect, because of transient delayed venous drainage compared with anterograde pedicle flaps and free flaps. For the muscle flap insetting, it is important to overlap muscle with the surrounding skin and imbricate the skin over the muscle to avoid

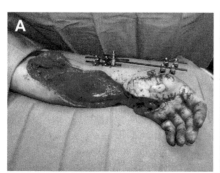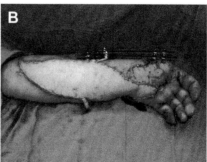

Fig. 14. (*A*) Complex injury of the left forearm with distal radius fracture, soft tissue loss, and exposed medium nerve. (*B*) Although the proximal portion of the forearm wound could have been covered with a skin graft over healthy muscle bellies, the entire wound was covered as a single aesthetic unit to provide better reconstructive homogeneity.

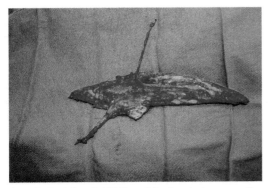

Fig. 15. Peripheral ALT flap thinning to improve flap insetting and decrease bulk. A 5-cm radius cuff of fascia is maintained to maximize blood supply to the flap.

any step-off deformities (**Fig. 15**). For small to moderate defects, a full-thickness skin graft covering the muscle flap can yield excellent cosmetic results. This thin full-thickness skin graft can be harvested from the overlying skin paddle of the muscle flap, which is discarded after skin graft harvest. This procedure also limits the morbidity to 1 single donor site.

SUMMARY

Optimal functional and aesthetic outcomes for hand reconstruction depend on optimizing the ideal flap for any given defect. This process needs to be truly individualized to be successful. Having a wider range of flap options in the armamentarium provides more flexibility in achieving these goals. The hand and reconstruction surgeon has to consider multiple factors before surgery and flap selection: patient body habitus, flap donor site options, and characteristics relative to the recipient site defect. Anatomic and functional variations should be taken into consideration in selecting the type of reconstruction. Local flaps provide reconstruction of the defects with like tissues and prevent additional morbidity to the other areas of the body. Adjuncts like primary donor site closure, suprafascial flap harvest, use of full-thickness skin grafting, and local rotation flaps can all improve the donor site closure and cosmesis. Extremity vascular status, tissue-texture match, and donor site morbidity should be taken into consideration when using a local flap. Free tissue transfer provides a wide variety of options for upper extremity reconstruction. Smaller defects, without exposed hardware, can be reconstructed with local intrinsic pedicle flaps, venous flaps, or fascial flaps with STSG. Larger defects with exposed hardware, or need for dead space

obliteration, require muscle or fasciocutaneous flaps for reconstruction. Muscle atrophy can be expected and often yields excellent cosmetic results, especially if muscle-sparing variants are used where the flap size is precisely tailored to the recipient size. This strategy also has the advantage of limiting donor site morbidity. Fasciocutaneous flaps frequently require revision surgery and debulking because of excess thickness. Having a greater availability of flap choices allows surgeons to be more selective in choosing the optimal fasciocutaneous flap donor site. The advent of freestyle perforator flaps, both free and pedicled, has played a larger role flap planning. Targeted debulking, redefining topographic regions by designing asymmetric skin excisions, and recreating natural creases that border adjacent aesthetic units may improve the aesthetic outcome. Attention to technical details during flap inset is critical. Measures such as peripheral flap thinning, recipient skin edge elevation and resection to healthy nonscarred tissue, meticulous inset for muscle flaps with proper overlap and native skin marsupialization may all improve the aesthetic outcomes after upper extremity reconstruction.

REFERENCES

1. Amadio PC, Wood MB, Cooney WP III, et al. Staged flexor tendon reconstruction in the fingers and hand. J Hand Surg Am 1988;13(4):559–62.
2. Brown DM, Upton J, Khouri RK. Free flap coverage of the hand. Clin Plast Surg 1997;24(1):57–62.
3. Elliott RA, Hoehn JG, Stayman JW. Management of the viable soft tissue cover in degloving injuries. Hand 1979;11(1):69–71.
4. Hsu WM, Wei FC, Lin CH, et al. The salvage of a degloved hand skin flap by arteriovenous shunting. Plast Reconstr Surg 1996;98(1):146–50.
5. Kozin SH, Thoder JJ, Lieberman G. Operative treatment of metacarpal and phalangeal shaft fractures. J Am Acad Orthop Surg 2000;8(2):111–21.
6. Nicolle FV, Woolhouse FM. Restoration of sensory function in severe degloving injuries of the hand. J Bone Joint Surg Am 1966;48(8):1511–8.
7. Scheker LR, Langley SJ, Martin DL, et al. Primary extensor tendon reconstruction in dorsal hand defects requiring free flaps. J Hand Surg 1993; 18(5):568–75.
8. Smith P, Jones M, Grobbelaar A. Two-stage grafting of flexor tendons: results after mobilisation by controlled early active movement. Scand J Plast Reconstr Surg Hand Surg 2004;38(4):220–7.
9. Swartz WM. Restoration of sensibility in mutilating hand injuries. Clin Plast Surg 1989;16(3):515–29.
10. Tajima T. Treatment of open crushing type of industrial injuries of the hand and forearm: degloving,

open circumferential, heat-press, and nail-bed injuries. J Trauma 1974;14(12):995–1011.

11. Weiland AJ, Villarreal-Rios A, Kleinert HE, et al. Replantation of digits and hands: analysis of surgical techniques and functional results in 71 patients with 86 replantations. Clin Orthop Relat Res 1978;(133):195–204.

12. Yildirim S, Taylan G, Eker G, et al. Free flap choice for soft tissue reconstruction of the severely damaged upper extremity. J Reconstr Microsurg 2006;22(8):599–609.

13. Friedrich JB, Katolik LI, Vedder NB. Soft tissue reconstruction of the hand. J Hand Surg Am 2009;34(6):1148–55.

14. Flugel A, Kehrer A, Heitmann C, et al. Coverage of soft-tissue defects of the hand with free fascial flaps. Microsurgery 2005;25(1):47–53.

15. Franceschi N, Yim KK, Lineaweaver WC, et al. Eleven consecutive combined latissimus dorsi and serratus anterior free muscle transplantations. Ann Plast Surg 1991;27(2):121–5.

16. Jones NF, Jarrahy R, Kaufman MR. Pedicled and free radial forearm flaps for reconstruction of the elbow, wrist, and hand. Plast Reconstr Surg 2008; 121(3):887–98.

17. Chen HC, Buchman MT, Wei FC. Free flaps for soft tissue coverage in the hand and fingers. Hand Clin 1999;15(4):541–54.

18. Upton J, Havlik RJ, Khouri RK. Refinements in hand coverage with microvascular free flaps. Clin Plast Surg 1992;19(4):841–57.

19. Carty MJ, Taghinia A, Upton J. Fascial flap reconstruction of the hand: a single surgeon's 30-year experience. Plast Reconstr Surg 2010;125(3): 953–62.

20. Giessler GA, Erdmann D, Germann G. Soft tissue coverage in devastating hand injuries. Hand Clin 2003;19(1):63–71, vi.

21. Talbot SG, Mehrara BJ, Disa JJ, et al. Soft-tissue coverage of the hand following sarcoma resection. Plast Reconstr Surg 2008;121(2):534–43.

22. Parrett BM, Bou-Merhi JS, Buntic RF, et al. Refining outcomes in dorsal hand coverage: consideration of aesthetics and donor-site morbidity. Plast Reconstr Surg 2010;126(5):1630–8.

23. Baumeister S, Menke H, Wittemann M, et al. Functional outcome after the Moberg advancement flap in the thumb. J Hand Surg Am 2002;27(1):105–14.

24. Chen C, Zhang X, Shao X, et al. Treatment of thumb tip degloving injury using the modified first dorsal metacarpal artery flap. J Hand Surg Am 2010;35(10):1663–70.

25. Logan A, Elliot D, Foucher G. Free toe pulp transfer to restore traumatic digital pulp loss. Br J Plast Surg 1985;38(4):497–500.

26. Shibata M, Iwabuchi Y, Kubota S, et al. Comparison of free and reversed pedicled posterior interosseous cutaneous flaps. Plast Reconstr Surg 1997;99(3): 791–802.

27. Brunelli F, Valenti P, Dumontier C, et al. The posterior interosseous reverse flap: experience with 113 flaps. Ann Plast Surg 2001;47(1):25–30.

28. Song R, Song Y, Yu Y. The upper arm free flap. Clin Plast Surg 1982;9(1):27–35.

29. Karamursel S, Bağdatli D, Markal N, et al. Versatility of the lateral arm free flap in various anatomic defect reconstructions. J Reconstr Microsurg 2005; 21(2):107–12.

30. Cronin TD. The cross finger flap: a new method of repair. Am Surg 1951;17(5):419–25.

31. Kappel DA, Burech JG. The cross-finger flap. An established reconstructive procedure. Hand Clin 1985;1(4):677–83.

32. Cohen BE, Cronin ED. An innervated cross-finger flap for fingertip reconstruction. Plast Reconstr Surg 1983;72(5):688–97.

33. Atasoy E, Ioakimidis E, Kasdan ML, et al. Reconstruction of the amputated finger tip with a triangular volar flap. A new surgical procedure. J Bone Joint Surg Am 1970;52(5):921–6.

34. Venkataswami R, Subramanian N. Oblique triangular flap: a new method of repair for oblique amputations of the fingertip and thumb. Plast Reconstr Surg 1980;66(2):296–300.

35. Evans DM, Martin DL. Step-advancement island flap for fingertip reconstruction. Br J Plast Surg 1988;41(2):105–11.

36. Joshi BB. A local dorsolateral island flap for restoration of sensation after avulsion injury of fingertip pulp. Plast Reconstr Surg 1974;54(2): 175–82.

37. Tranquilli L. Ricostruzione dell'apice delle falangi unguali median autoplastica volare peduncolata per socorrimento. Inform Trauma Lavoro 1935;1: 186–93 [in Italian].

38. Lai CS, Lin SD, Yang CC. The reverse digital artery flap for fingertip reconstruction. Ann Plast Surg 1989;22(6):495–500.

39. Kojima T, Tsuchida Y, Hirasé Y, et al. Reverse vascular pedicle digital island flap. Br J Plast Surg 1990;43(3):290–5.

40. Page R, Chang J. Reconstruction of hand soft-tissue defects: alternatives to the radial forearm fasciocutaneous flap. J Hand Surg Am 2006; 31(5):847–56.

41. Pederson WC, Stevanovic M, Zalavras C, et al. Reconstructive surgery: extensive injuries to the upper limb. In: Mathes SJ, editor. Plastic surgery, vol. 7, 2nd edition. Philadelphia: Saunders; 2006. p. 317–49.

42. Brooks D, Buntic RF. Partial muscle harvest: our first 100 cases attempting to preserve form and function at the donor site. Microsurgery 2008; 28(8):606–11.

43. Buntic RF, Brooks D. Free partial medial rectus muscle flap for closure of complex extremity wounds. Plast Reconstr Surg 2005;116(5):1434–7.

44. Fassio E, Laulan J, Aboumoussa J, et al. Serratus anterior free fascial flap for dorsal hand coverage. Ann Plast Surg 1999;43(1):77–82.

45. Lee N, Roh S, Yang K, et al. Reconstruction of hand and forearm after sarcoma resection using antero-lateral thigh free flap. J Plast Reconstr Aesthet Surg 2009;62(12):e584–6.

46. Ulusal BG, Lin YT, Ulusal AE, et al. Free lateral arm flap for 1-stage reconstruction of soft tissue and composite defects of the hand: a retrospective analysis of 118 cases. Ann Plast Surg 2007;58(2): 173–8.

47. Gatti JE, LaRossa D, Brousseau DA, et al. Assessment of neovascularization and timing of flap division. Plast Reconstr Surg 1984;73(3):396–402.

48. Farber GL, Taylor KF, Smith AC. Pedicled thoracoabdominal flap coverage about the elbow in traumatic war injuries. Hand 2010;5(1):43–8.

49. Flatt AE. The thenar flap. J Bone Joint Surg Br 1957;39-B(1):80–5.

50. Heng D, Zhang C, Yao Y, et al. Experimental study on early division of cross-finger pedicle flap and its clinical application. Chin J Traumatol 2000;3(3): 159–62.

51. McGrath MH, Adelberg D, Finseth F. The intravenous fluorescein test: use in timing of groin flap division. J Hand Surg Am 1979;4(1):19–22.

52. Higgins JP, Seruya M. Visual subunits of the hand: proposed guidelines for revision surgery after flap reconstruction of the traumatized hand. J Reconstr Microsurg 2011;27(9):551–7.

53. Richardson D, Fisher SE, Vaughan ED, et al. Radial forearm flap donor-site complications and morbidity: a prospective study. Plast Reconstr Surg 1997;99(1):109–15.

54. Agostini T, Russo GL, Zhang YX, et al. Adipofascial anterolateral thigh flap safety: applications and complications. Arch Plast Surg 2013;40(2):91–6.

55. Lin TS, Jeng SF, Chiang YC. Resurfacing with full-thickness skin graft after debulking procedure for bulky flap of the hand. J Trauma 2008;65(1): 123–6.

56. Chang J, Jones N. Muscle free flaps with full-thickness skin grafting: improved contour over traditional musculocutaneous free flaps. Microsurgery 2001;21(2):70–3.

57. Schwabegger AH, Harpf C, Rainer C. Muscle-sparing latissimus dorsi myocutaneous flap with maintenance of muscle innervation, function, and aesthetic appearance of the donor site. Plast Reconstr Surg 2003;111(4):1407–11.

58. Tan O, Algan S, Denktas Kuduban S, et al. Versatile use of the muscle and nerve sparing latissimus dorsi flap. Microsurgery 2012;32(2):103–10.

59. Colohan S, Wong C, Lakhiani C, et al. The free descending branch muscle-sparing latissimus dorsi flap: vascular anatomy and clinical applications. Plast Reconstr Surg 2012;130(6):776e–87e.

60. Walle L, Vollbach FH, Fansa H. Arterialized venous free flaps for resurfacing hand and finger defects. Handchir Mikrochir Plast Chir 2013;45(3):160–6 [in German].

61. Trovato MJ, Brooks D, Buntic RF, et al. Simultaneous coverage of two separate dorsal digital defects with a syndactylizing venous free flap. Microsurgery 2008;28(4):248–51.

62. Woo SH, Kim KC, Lee GJ, et al. A retrospective analysis of 154 arterialized venous flaps for hand reconstruction: an 11-year experience. Plast Reconstr Surg 2007;119(6):1823–38.

63. Brooks D. The "reliably unreliable" venous flap. J Hand Surg Am 2009;34(7):1361–2 [author reply: 1362].

Dermal Skin Substitutes for Upper Limb Reconstruction
Current Status, Indications, and Contraindications

Shady A. Rehim, MB ChB, MSc, MRCS[a],
Maneesh Singhal, MBBS, MS, MCh[b],
Kevin C. Chung, MD, MS[c],*

KEYWORDS

- Dermal skin substitutes • Integra • Matriderm • Reconstruction • Trauma • Upper extremity

KEY POINTS

- The provision of skin coverage for the upper extremity presents surgeons with several challenges. The special functional and physiologic requirements of the integument such as mobility and sensibility need special consideration when performing soft issue reconstructions of the upper limb.
- Adhering to the concept of the reconstructive ladder, soft tissue reconstruction of the upper extremity has treatment options that range from the application of skin grafts to reconstruction with microsurgical free tissue transfer. Dermal skin substitutes have been applied recently as part of the reconstructive ladder to expand the reconstructive options.
- Common clinical indications of dermal skin substitutes in the upper extremity include management of burns and soft tissue coverage of traumatic injuries with exposed tendons, joints, and bones. Other clinical uses may involve resurfacing of wounds following tumor resection, excision of Dupuytren cords, and repair of congenital hand deformities (eg, skin coverage following syndactyly release).
- Common associated complications of dermal skin substitutes are infection, hematoma, graft failure, and the need for multiple procedures. One should consider whether the cost of dermal skin substitute justify its use and the stiffness of the hand that results from the required long period of immobility to assure vascularization.

INTRODUCTION

The first recorded application of skin substitutes (xenografts) dates back to the 15th century BC as mentioned in the Papyrus of Ebers.[1] In 1981 Yannas[2] and Burke[3] developed artificial skin substitutes, a dermal regeneration template composed of a bilayer of temporary silicone epidermis and a

Disclosure: None of the authors has a financial interest in any of the products, devices, or drugs mentioned in this article. Supported in part by grants from the National Institute of Arthritis and Musculoskeletal and Skin Diseases and National Institute on Aging (R01 AR062066), the National Institute of Arthritis and Musculoskeletal and Skin Diseases (2R01 AR047328-06), and a Midcareer Investigator Award in Patient-Oriented Research (K24 AR053120) (Dr K.C. Chung). Dr M. Singhal has received a fellowship grant from Indian Council of Medical Research, New Delhi, India to study various applications of skin substitutes.

[a] Section of Plastic Surgery, Department of Surgery, University of Michigan Health System, Ann Arbor, MI, USA; [b] Department of Surgical Disciplines, All India Institute of Medical Sciences (AIMS), New Delhi, India; [c] Section of Plastic Surgery, University of Michigan Medical School, University of Michigan Health System, 2130 Taubman Center, SPC 5340, 1500 East Medical Center Drive, Ann Arbor, MI 48109-5340, USA
* Corresponding author.
E-mail address: kecchung@umich.edu

Hand Clin 30 (2014) 239–252
http://dx.doi.org/10.1016/j.hcl.2014.02.001

porous collagen-chondroitin 6-sulfate fibrillar dermis, for the treatment of acute extensive burns. Eventually, upper limb surgeons expanded the use of these skin substitutes to cover areas as small as the fingertips.[4]

Soft tissue repair of the upper extremity has traditionally followed the hierarchy of the reconstructive ladder that progresses from simple methods of wound closure such as the application of skin grafts to more sophisticated methods of free tissue transfer. Over the past 2 decades, technological innovations, especially in tissue engineering, have introduced other viable alternatives for the provision of skin coverage, remarkably biosynthetic materials such as dermal skin substitutes. When dermal skin substitutes are used in conjunction with a skin graft, the resulting skin is of better quality, thickness, and pliability than reconstructions using only split-thickness skin grafts.[5] Furthermore, dermal substitutes can be used in the hand to cover critical structures such as tendons devoid of paratenon, cartilage without perichondrium, and bone without periosteum. The full biointegration of dermal substitutes requires a well-vascularized wound bed that is clear of infection. Thus in potentially contaminated devascularized wounds, autologous tissue transfer is more appropriate. However there are numerous clinical situations in which dermal skin substitutes would offer the upper limb surgeon an additional reconstructive option in solving difficult problems whereby local tissue is damaged or not available. The term, "dermal skin substitutes," is commonly used to refer to a wide range of products that are currently available on the market.[6] In this article the terms dermal skin substitutes, dermal substitutes, dermal matrices, and dermal regeneration template are used interchangeably to refer to several types of skin substitutes that have been commonly reported in the soft tissue reconstructions of the upper extremity.

HISTOLOGIC PROPERTIES OF DERMAL SKIN SUBSTITUTES

Dermal skin substitutes are a heterogeneous group of wound coverage materials that aids in wound closure and replaces some of the functions of the skin, either temporarily or permanently, depending on the product characteristics.[7] They provide several biologic and physiologic properties of human dermis that allow and/or promote new tissue growth and optimize the conditions for healing.

These biodegradable materials are composed of a bilayer of collagen and glycosaminoglycan covered by a temporary epidermal substitute.[8]

The porous matrix applied to the wound bed acts as a scaffold for the in-growth of the host's fibroblasts, endothelial cells, and endogenous collagen that subsequently vascularizes and creates a distinct layer called the "neodermis."[9] Contrary to skin grafts, dermal matrices are independent of imbibition or inosculation for immediate viability. In addition, they invoke minimal inflammatory or immunologic response owing to their acellular composition.[8] Moiemen and colleagues[9] described 4 distinct histologic phases of integration of one type of dermal substitutes (**Table 1**), based on histologic specimens obtained from sites of soft tissue repaired with dermal substitutes. In another study, the same group analyzed specimens obtained more than 2 years from sites reconstructed with dermal skin substitutes. They found that the newly formed collagen and elastin consist of an abnormal morphology that does not resemble normal skin collagen. Nevertheless, they reported good clinical outcomes in terms of decreased scarring, skin pliability, and acceptable patient satisfaction. In addition, for the first time they reported the presence of nerve fibers within the reticular (deep) dermis,[10] suggesting that a gradual regeneration process of nerve endings occur within the dermal regeneration template, a finding that correlated with improvement of sensory function among patients involved in their study. On the other hand, adnexal structures such as sweat glands or hair follicles have not

Table 1		
Four stages of dermal skin substitute integration within host tissue as described by Moiemen and colleagues		
Histologic Stage	**Duration**	**Sequence of Events**
Imbibition	Minutes	Dermal substitutes start to adhere to wound bed
Fibroblast migration	Day 7	Fibroblasts start collagen secretion
Neovascularization	Day 14	Neovascularization (formation of new blood vessels)
Remodeling and maturation	Day 28	Host collagen replaces the dermal collagen matrix

Data from Moiemen NS, Vlachou E, Staiano JJ, et al. Reconstructive surgery with Integra dermal regeneration template: histologic study, clinical evaluation, and current practice. Plast Reconstr Surg 2006;117(Suppl 7):160S–74S.

been observed to grow within the newly formed dermis.[10] Finally, the authors concluded that beyond a 2-year period, the dermal matrix is completely replaced by native collagen and no long-term residual template matrix can be found within the examined specimens, a property that maintains the biodegradable nature of these dermal substitutes.

APPLICATION OF DERMAL SUBSTITUTES

The mainstay of management of upper extremity wounds is centered on the adequate surgical debridement of wounds followed by early soft tissue coverage and mobilization. Following debridement, dermal skin substitutes can be used to cover the resultant defect. Although the composition of different dermal regeneration templates is slightly different, their method of application and uses is principally similar. Nevertheless, one must always follow the manufacturer's instructions for each type of dermal regeneration template used.

The first step requires the assessment of wound vascularity. The amount of vascularized tissue for the successful incorporation of dermal substitutes is not well defined.[11] Whether the wound is eligible to be covered by a dermal matrix or not is therefore left to the surgeon's judgment and experience. Irradiated wounds or wounds with extensive devitalized tissue are not suitable for coverage with dermal skin substitutes. Another important factor for the successful take of dermal matrices includes the presence or absence of infection. Heimbach and colleagues[12] reported a 26% less take in infected versus noninfected sites. Moreover, Shirley and colleagues[13] reported a case of a fatal toxic shock syndrome whereby the dermal substitute grafted site was colonized with methicillin-resistant *Staphylococcus aureus*. For these reasons it is strongly recommended that clear bacteriology cultures of the wounds be obtained before the application of dermal substitutes.

Once the wound is deemed suitable for coverage, the dermal matrix is applied and secured along the rim of the defect in a similar fashion to a skin graft. The dermal matrix should be applied as adherent as possible to the wound bed. Any fluid collection, air bubbles, or folding of the template could intervene between the inner surface of the dermal matrix and the wound bed, and consequently, may result in graft failure. Some surgeons may mesh dermal substitutes similar to skin grafts to increase the surface area covered by the dermal substitutes and allow fluid extravasation (eg, hematoma or seroma).

However, the authors advocate the use of unmeshed dermal substitutes whenever possible to fill the void, which decrease the possibility of recurrent skin contractures and improve the final aesthetic appearance of the grafted site (**Fig. 1**). Dermal regeneration templates that are currently available require either single-staged or 2-staged reconstructions. The single-stage procedure applies the dermal matrix covered with a skin graft in one procedure, whereas the latter involves the application of the dermal matrix followed by coverage with a skin graft 5 to 7 days later to allow for vascularization of the regeneration template. Typically a split-thickness skin graft setting of 0.011 to 0.015 inch is used to cover the dermal matrix. Although the successful take of full-thickness skin grafts over dermal substitutes has been reported in small-sized wounds over the digits, the greater metabolic demand of full-thickness skin grafts makes them prone to ischemia and necrosis and is therefore discouraged.[14]

Following the application of dermal substitutes, simple nonadhesive dressings are used to cover the wound site. Negative pressure wound therapy/dressing has been used to stabilize dermal substitutes to prevent shearing forces and minimize development of hematoma and seroma. It has also been postulated that the application of negative pressure wound therapy/dressing may improve the take of composite dermal substitutes and skin grafts by stimulating angiogenesis, increasing cell proliferation, and enhancing vascularization of the regeneration template. However, the current evidence derived from a randomized control trial and histologic studies does not support this assumption.[15,16]

CLINICAL INDICATIONS AND OUTCOMES OF DERMAL SKIN SUBSTITUTES

Dermal skin substitutes have been commonly used in acute and chronic reconstructive burn surgery. The US Food and Drug Administration more recently extended the indications of dermal skin substitutes to include non-burn-related, traumatic, and chronic extremity wounds.[17] Furthermore, these medical devices have been proposed as part of the surgeon's reconstructive ladder (**Fig. 2**).[5] However, the role of dermal substitutes in upper limb reconstruction is still evolving. Apart from burn surgery, there is no clear guidance on the exact indications of these medical devices for several reasons. First, wounds of the upper extremity have various causes and patients often have different comorbidities. Second, the current available evidence is mostly composed of

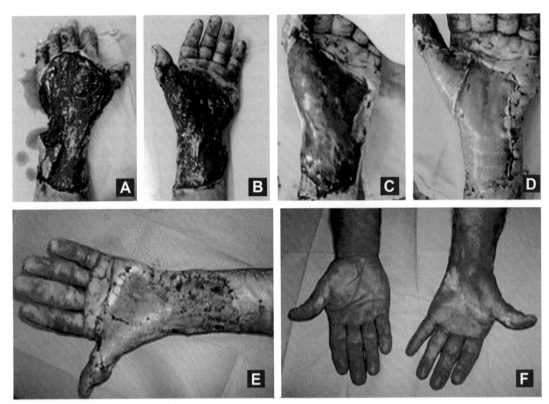

Fig. 1. Reconstruction of an extensive avulsion injury of the upper extremity with dermal skin substitutes. The dermal matrix should be applied on a vascular bed after wound debridement and secured to wound edges (A–C). A sheet of single-stage dermal matrix was applied to the wound and covered directly with a skin graft in one procedure (D). Complete take of the composite dermal substitute and skin graft 1 week after surgery (E), and good postoperative results at 2-year follow-up (F). However, when using a 2-stage dermal substitute, the regeneration template should be placed with the silicone side up. After 2 to 3 weeks, the silicone layer is peeled off and covered with a skin graft (not shown in this image). (*From* Demiri E, Papaconstantinou A, Dionyssiou A, et al. Reconstruction of skin avulsion injuries of the upper extremity with Integra® dermal regeneration template and skin grafts in a single-stage procedure. Arch Orthop Trauma Surg 2013;133(11):1523; with kind permission from Springer Science and Business Media.)

noncomparative retrospective case series and individual surgeons' experience. Therefore, evaluating the effectiveness of dermal substitutes and their long-term functional outcomes in the overall wound healing of the extremity is difficult to interpret.

Another area of concern is cost associated with dermal substitutes. Aside from clinical effectiveness, costs need to be evaluated to assess the benefits of a new treatment comprehensively. Within the current global economic uncertainties, the high initial purchase cost of dermal substitutes may prove a disincentive to health care commissioners and purchasing bodies that may limit their availability to surgeons and patients; this is particularly true in developing countries, where economically privileged countries are more likely to afford the use dermal skin substitutes. To date, there is a single cost analysis study that compared the total costs involved with dermal substitutes

reconstructions versus total costs of skin graft–only reconstructions for the treatment of small-sized burns. Although the total costs among the dermal substitutes group culminated higher expenses per patient (2218 Euros), this was not significantly higher than the skin graft–only group (1703 Euros).[18] Interestingly, indirect health-related costs such as length of hospital stay and overheads were found to be the most important factors influencing the total cost of treatment. The decision to use dermal substitutes may therefore be a clinical one. A major limitation of this study was the limited follow-up period of 12 months. The costs of further reconstructive surgeries or revisions were not considered. Thus it is imperative that further cost-effectiveness studies with longer follow-up are conducted to justify the use of dermal substitutes and help in resource allocation. Last, surgeon's experience and patient preferences should also be considered in the final

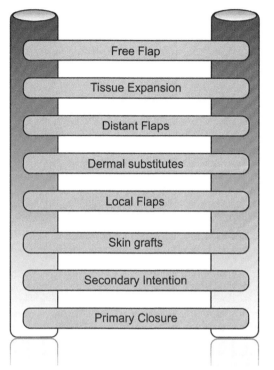

Fig. 2. Modification of the reconstructive ladder incorporating dermal skin substitutes. (*Adapted from* Janis JE, Kwon RK, Attinger CE. The new reconstructive ladder: modifications to the traditional model. Plast Reconstr Surg 2011;127(Suppl 1):205S–12S; with permission.)

decision-making process. Nonetheless, dermal skin substitutes have been used in all of the following with various degrees of success.

Burn Injuries

The upper extremities and especially the hands are among the most commonly affected areas of the body with burn injuries. Burns of these special areas are considered severe, because even a small wound may cause profound functional disability. In addition, in regions with requirements of elasticity, pliability, and mobility such as the axilla, elbow, wrist, and hand regions, it is important to replace burnt areas with skin of similar characteristics to the native tissue to preserve the range of motion and consequently the limb function. Current indications of dermal skin substitutes include both acute (eg, deep partial or full-thickness burns, **Figs. 3** and **4**) and chronic burns (eg, hypertrophic scars and scar contractures). Autologous skin grafts have been traditionally used for the provision of skin coverage following debridement of burns. However, the resultant aesthetic disfigurement, development of adherent scars, and recurrent scar contractures may require revision surgeries to enhance aesthetics and restore the function and mobility of the affected parts.

A prospective controlled trial of patients with bilateral acute full-thickness burns located on the dorsum of the hand was conducted to evaluate the effectiveness of dermal substitutes in treating

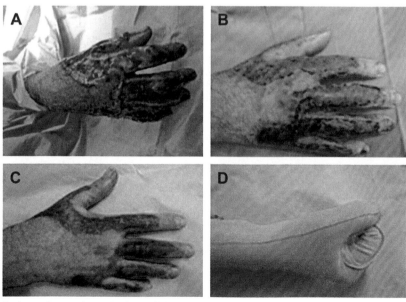

Fig. 3. A full-thickness burn of the dorsum of the hand and fingers (*A, B*). Two weeks after split-thickness skin graft over the neodermis and elastic compression therapy (*C, D*). (*From* Cuadra A, Correa G, Roa R, et al. Functional results of burned hands treated with Integra. J Plast Reconstr Aesthet Surg 2012;65(2):231; with permission.)

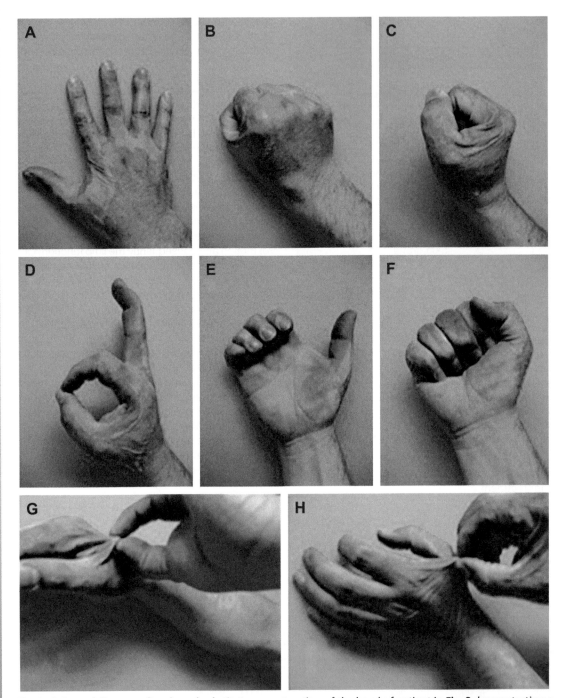

Fig. 4. A 6-year follow-up after dermal substitute reconstruction of the hand of patient in **Fig. 3** demonstrating a good range of motion (*A–F*). Pliability of the skin in the unburned hand (*G*) compared with pliability of the skin in the burned hand treated with skin substitute (*H*). (*From* Cuadra A, Correa G, Roa R, et al. Functional results of burned hands treated with Integra. J Plast Reconstr Aesthet Surg 2012;65(2):232; with permission.)

such a common injury.[19] Intraindividual comparison was performed by treating one hand with composite dermal substitutes and skin grafts (intervention), and the contralateral hand was treated using the traditional method of burn

excision and skin grafting (control). A total of 18 patients were included and a single-staged dermal regeneration template was used in this study. Assessors were blinded to the intervention and control groups. Outcomes measures are wound site evaluation of dermal substitutes and skin graft take, need for re-grafting, skin elasticity assessed by Vancouver Burn Skin Score, and range of motion assessed by measuring the Finger-Tip-Palmar-Crease-Distance and Finger-Nail-Table-Distance of the index to small fingers. The results of this study showed no significant difference between the 2 groups regarding dermal substitute or skin graft take or the need for regrafting. However, hands treated with the dermal regeneration template were superior to skin-grafted-only wounds in skin elasticity and active range of motion. The use of a single-staged regeneration template allows early institution of physical therapy once the composite graft is deemed stable, a process that usually takes 5 to 7 days. However, if a 2-stage dermal regeneration template is used, the hand could be immobilized for up to 2 weeks before a skin graft can be applied to the dermal matrix, which may increase the risk of joint stiffness. Several other reports have shown similar results using dermal substitutes for treating acute and chronic burns on the hands and digits.[20–23]

Contracture release and scar resurfacing using dermal substitutes have also been reported in the upper extremity, such as in skin contractures around the axilla and elbow joint. Skin contractures of these regions are notoriously difficult to treat and often result in severe restriction of movement that prevents patients from performing functions of daily living such as the ability to eat, shower, or drive independently. Conventionally, the treatment of these skin contractures included either scar lengthening procedures by the means of multiple Z-plasties or scar excision and resurfacing with skin grafts, fasciocutaneous flaps, or recruitment of adjacent skin after a period of tissue expansion. A multicenter study of 13 study centers in the United States, France, Germany, and the United Kingdom was conducted to evaluate the outcomes of contracture release procedures incorporating a dermal regeneration template for 89 consecutive patients who underwent a total of 127 contracture releases.[24] Thirty-nine of the treated contractures were located at the axilla and elbow regions. Postoperatively, the most commonly observed complication was wound infection followed by fluid collection underneath the regeneration template, such as a seroma or hematoma. In regards to recurrence of skin contractures, this was not observed during the duration of the follow-up period of the study that extended for 11 months. Physician ratings of contracture release outcomes in range of motion or function were rated good to excellent in 75% of the cases. Patient-reported outcomes showed that 82% of the patients were satisfied with

postoperative range of motion, aesthetic appearance, and pain relief. Despite these encouraging results, the findings of this study should be interpreted with caution due to the relatively short postoperative follow-up period that can be considered a limitation, because wounds may take up to 24 months to form mature scars or recurrence of contracture.

Traumatic Injuries

Traumatic high-energy shearing forces cause disruption of tissue planes that often result in skin avulsions and degloving injuries. The advantages of early wound coverage are well recognized by minimizing infection and preventing tissue desiccation as well as allowing patients' early rehabilitation and mobilization. Based on wound characteristics and structures affected, these injury patterns are conventionally treated by debridement of devitalized tissues followed by provision of adequate soft tissue coverage. Wounds with exposed tendons and bones are not suitable for skin graft coverage. Regional or distant flap transfers can be appropriate alternatives; however, coexistence of multiple injuries or substantial patients' morbidity may preclude patients from undergoing lengthy flap procedures. Dermal skin substitutes can be thought of in these circumstances as either a temporary or a permanent method of wound coverage (see **Fig. 1**; **Fig. 5**).

The ultimate goal of any reconstructive procedure is the resumption of normal activities of the affected limb as fast as possible to avoid joint

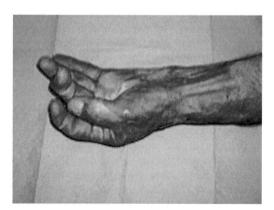

Fig. 5. A 2-year follow-up of the patient in **Fig. 1**, demonstrating good pinch grip of the thumb. (*From* Demiri E, Papaconstantinou A, Dionyssiou A, et al. Reconstruction of skin avulsion injuries of the upper extremity with Integra® dermal regeneration template and skin grafts in a single-stage procedure. Arch Orthop Trauma Surg 2013;133(11):1521–6; with kind permission from Springer Science and Business Media.)

stiffness and disuse atrophy. For soft tissue reconstruction, most of published work have assessed the success of dermal substitutes based on their ability of successful integration and provision of definitive closure of the defect. However, optimizing hand function following complex injury requires a stable and durable soft tissue coverage that can withstand secondary surgeries to address underlying deformities. Thus far, the possibility of performing secondary corrective surgery at a site that has been previously reconstructed with dermal substitutes has not been investigated. Furthermore, despite the good skin elasticity and pliability of wound sites reconstructed with dermal substitutes, these biodegradable materials do not replace like with like. Tissue replaced with dermal skin substitutes lacks essential components of normal skin such as sweat gland and hair follicles. In addition, restoration of sensibility is suboptimal. These considerations are all important especially when reconstructing tissue over the palm of the hand or volar surface of the digits where the hand function can be greatly affected if replaced with tissue of a less quality or that does not resemble normal skin characteristics. Local flaps, if available, are considered the treatment of choice to repair small-to-medium sized soft tissue defects. For larger defects the wound extent and the need for functional repair should be addressed first. The comparative effectiveness of dermal substitutes and skin graft to flap surgery has yet to be shown. However, in an isolated soft tissue defect, whether the reconstruction should be performed using dermal skin substitutes or autologous tissue transfer should be evaluated on a case-by-case basis (**Table 2**) after taking into account a myriad of considerations including structures affected, patient's comorbidities, patient's preference, surgeon's skills, and length of limb immobilization.

Only a few studies and case reports have been published so far whereby surgeons used dermal skin substitutes for immediate wound coverage after traumatic injuries.[25,26] Graham and colleagues[27] reported 5 patients with severe degloving injuries of the upper extremity who were treated with dermal skin substitutes. The surface area of reconstructed areas ranged from 50 to 1000 cm^2 and 90% of the patients sustained underlying open fractures. Soft tissue reconstruction of these defects was achieved by means of composite dermal substitutes and split-thickness skin grafts. The wounds were first debrided the same day as the injury and then were covered with negative pressure therapy temporarily. After the wounds were deemed viable and clear of infection, dermal substitutes were applied at a median of 14 days and skin grafts were placed at a median of

27 days after injury, respectively. At a 5-month follow-up, all patients had a complete skin graft taken and no contractures or other graft-related complications were noted that required revision or limited return to normal function. In another series, Taras and colleagues[28] treated 21 traumatic finger injuries resulting in soft tissue loss with exposed underlying bone, joints, hardware, and tendons with dermal skin substitutes and full-thickness skin grafts (**Fig. 6**). All patients received 2 operations that were spaced 3 weeks apart. The first procedure required wound debridement and application of the skin substitute followed by a second procedure that covered the wound with dermal skin substitute and full-thickness skin grafts. Patients were followed up for 12 months. The wounds reconstructed ranged from 1 to 24 cm^2, while the largest single area covered with dermal substitutes was 12 cm^2. Complete graft-take was reported in 16 (80%) digits and partial graft loss was reported in 4 (20%) digits. However, no further treatment was required and most patients were able to return to their employment. Dermal regeneration templates have also been used in a "stacked" fashion to increase the thickness and durability of coverage over exposed bone and tendons.[29] One should be cautious using these different applications of dermal substitutes that may considerably increase the duration of treatment and immobilization of the hand that may result in further problems such as hand stiffness.

OTHER POTENTIAL INDICATIONS OF DERMAL SUBSTITUTES
Soft Tissue Reconstruction After Tumor Resection

Tumor resection and wide local excision may leave patients with defects requiring complex reconstructive surgery. The reconstructive approach following tumor resection differs greatly from the traditional approach of soft tissue reconstruction resulting from other mentioned causes, for several reasons. First, the treatment of suspected benign tumors (eg, pyogenic granuloma or a soft tissue lipoma) is usually achieved by a direct excision of the lesion and skin closure. However, in suspected malignant tumors such as basal cell carcinoma, squamous cell carcinoma, or malignant melanoma, a resection margin of healthy adjacent tissue is usually required that would necessitate some form of a soft tissue reconstruction to close the resultant defect. Second, different types of tumors require different treatment and, without formal histopathology results, it is difficult for the surgeon to predict the actual size and extent of the final defect that need to be reconstructed.

Table 2
Summary of different features of soft tissue reconstructive techniques of the upper extremity

Method of Reconstruction	Different Characteristics of Various Methods of Soft-Tissue Reconstruction								
	Coverage of Bare Tendons, Bone, and Joints[a]	Size of Defect Coverage	Skin Quality	Sensory Recovery[b]	Number of Procedures Required[c]	Mean Duration of Postoperative Limb Immobilization Required (d)	Level of Difficulty	Donor-Site Deformity	Cost
Split-thickness skin graft	No	Small- to large-sized defects	Average	No	Single	7–10	Easy to perform	Yes	$
Full-thickness skin graft	No	Small defects	Good	No	Single	7–10	Easy to perform	Yes (minimal scarring)	$
Dermal substitutes	Yes	Small- to large-sized defects	Good–very good	Suboptimal recovery	One to 2 procedures depending on the use of a single- or two-stage dermal substitute	7–21[d]	Easy to perform. However, there is a learning curve to perform satisfactorily	No	$$$$
Local flaps	Yes	Small defects	Excellent	Yes	One or 2 procedures depends on type of flap used	7	Average difficulty	Yes (minimal scarring)	$
Pedicled and regional flaps	Yes	Small- to large-sized defects	Very good	No	Two or more	21	Average difficulty	Yes	$$
Microvascular free flaps	Yes	Large-sized defects	Very good	No	Usually single but may require revision procedures	7	Difficult, requires adequate expertise and training to achieve good results	Yes (muscle flaps> fasciocutaneous flaps)	$$$

[a] Tendons, bones, and cartilage without paratenon, periosteum, and perichondrium.
[b] Not including specialized sensation of the palm of the hand.
[c] Not including secondary or revision surgery.
[d] Single-stage dermal substitutes requires shorter period of limb immobilization.

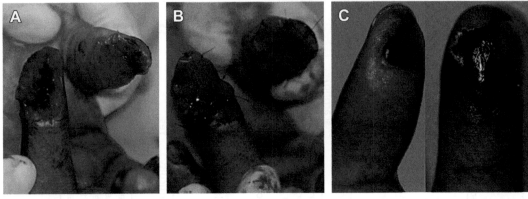

Fig. 6. (*A–C*) Demonstrating an amputation injury of the thumb and ring fingers successfully covered by dermal regeneration template. (*From* Taras JS, Sapienza A, Roach JB, et al. Acellular dermal regeneration template for soft tissue reconstruction of the digits. J Hand Surg Am 2010;35(3):417–18; with permission.)

Conventionally, skin grafts or locoregional flaps have been used to cover defects following tumor resection in the hand and upper extremity. However, skin grafts are prone to contraction, leave a contour defect, and are less robust, especially when used to cover previously irradiated wound beds. Locoregional flaps offer superior results than skin grafts because they provide tissue of similar texture, color, and thickness. Nevertheless, the disadvantage of reconstructing soft tissue defects following tumor excision with local or regional flaps is the limited ability to monitor disease recurrence of the reconstructed area.

Dermal skin substitutes may be a reasonable alternative for soft tissue reconstruction following tumor resection. They can act as a temporizing reconstruction while awaiting formal histology. They do not result in changes that may not be reversible and may also be the only treatment needed (**Figs. 7** and **8**). This application of dermal substitutes is particularly useful in elderly patients and patients deemed of a higher anesthetic risk. Chalmers and colleagues[30] successfully treated 5 patients using dermal skin substitutes and skin grafts following excision of squamous cell carcinoma and malignant melanoma from the digits. A

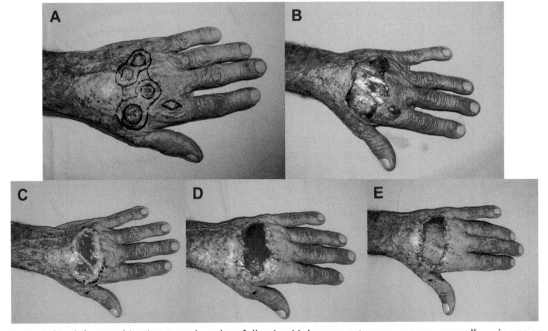

Fig. 7. A skin defect resulting in exposed tendons following Mohs surgery to remove squamous cell carcinoma on the dorsum of the hand (*A, B*). The defect primarily covered with dermal skin substitute (*C*). Two weeks later, a sheet of split-thickness skin graft was applied (*D, E*).

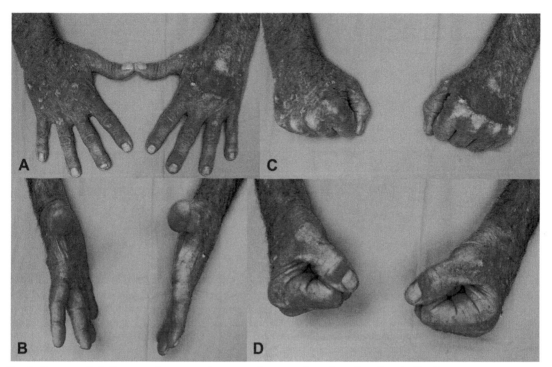

Fig. 8. One-month follow-up, demonstrating a good range of motion of patient in **Fig. 7**.

100% graft take and full range of motion were achieved in most patients. Only a few case reports are currently available that discuss the role of dermal substitutes to reconstruct skin defects following tumors resection.[31–33]

Soft Tissue Reconstruction After Radial Forearm Flap Harvest

Although the radial forearm flap is regarded as a workhorse flap in reconstructive surgery, the aesthetic and functional morbidity of the donor-site remain a considerable concern. Donor-site repair of the radial forearm flap has been usually achieved by either split-thickness or full-thickness skin grafts. These methods may result in complications such as tendon exposure, decreased sensation, functional disability (including limited hand mobility and decreased strength), and poor aesthetic appearance. Harvesting a suprafascial radial forearm flap[34–37] may help to minimize these complications, but not every surgeon is well versed with this technique. To date, there is no consensus on the best way of closing radial forearm flap defects. Several authors have used dermal substitutes to cover radial forearm defects with satisfactory results (**Fig. 9**).[35,36] Murray and colleagues[38] repaired radial forearm free flap donor sites in 29 patients using composite dermal substitutes and ultrathin split-thickness skin grafts. Full healing

was achieved within 4 to 6 weeks with negligible donor-site complications, excellent aesthetics, and minimal scar contracture. Gravvanis and colleagues[39] applied the same technique as Murray in 6 patients following suprafacial radial forearm free flap harvest. After 24 days, the donor site demonstrated complete wound healing. After 9 months, all patients had normal range of motion of the wrist and the fingers, normal power grip, and power pinch. Finally, Medina and colleagues[40] used a 2-stage novel approach to improve aesthetics of radial forearm free flap donor sites using dermal substitutes. In the first stage, the dermal matrix was implanted in the forearm for 2 weeks. In the second stage, skin flaps are raised superficial to the dermal matrix and then the radial forearm tissue along with dermal matrix is harvested on the vascular pedicle (as a prefabricated flap). The forearm skin flaps are then reflected back to cover the defect.

Soft Tissue Reconstruction After Excision of Dupuytren Contracture

Dupuytren disease is a fibroproliferative disorder of unclear cause that often results in shortening and thickening of the palmar fascia, leading to permanent and irreversible flexion contracture of the digits. In severe or recurrent disease, a dermofasciectomy may be required. Dermofasciectomy

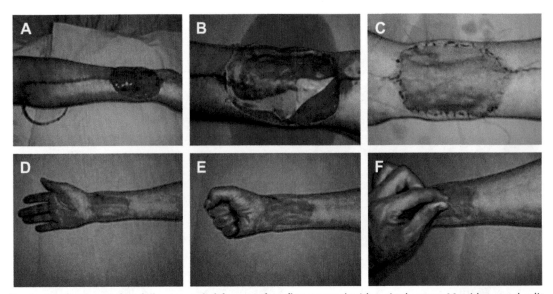

Fig. 9. A soft tissue defect following radial forearm free flap covered with a single-stage Matriderm and split-thickness skin graft (*A–C*). At 12-month follow-up, skin cover demonstrating good pliability and normal range 1305 of motion of the hand (*D–F*). (*From* Haslik W, Kamolz LP, Mann F, et al. Management of full-thickness skin defects in the hand and wrist region: first long-term experiences with the dermal matrix Matriderm. J Plast Reconstr Aesthet Surg 2010:63(2):363; with permission.)

involves the removal of diseased palmar fascia (cord and nodule) and overlying affected skin, and a full-thickness skin graft is usually required to cover the resultant defect. Alternatively, a skin substitute without a skin graft can be placed over these defects that would eventually heal by epithelialization process and spare the patient from creating a donor site. So far, the use of dermal matrices with Dupuytren disease has been limited to a single case report. Ellis and Kulber[41] reported a patient with severe recurrent Dupuytren contracture of the palm extending to the small finger that underwent prior failed needle aponeurectomy and palmar fasciectomy and resulted in severe flexion contracture and functional loss of the digit. Following excision of the cord and skin, a defect measuring 14 cm^2 was resurfaced with a dermal regeneration template. After a 2-year follow-up period, the patient demonstrated a substantial improvement of range of motion of the finger and no signs of recurrence of the disease. Although this technique may sound promising, further studies on histologic evidence regarding disease progression and recurrence are required to support a wider application of this treatment modality.

SUMMARY

Tissue repair with dermal skin substitutes seems to be a useful tool in reconstructive surgery. The immediate skin coverage achieved using dermal substitutes consists of a reconstructive option for managing injuries of the upper extremity that minimizes donor-site morbidity and provides final acceptable functional and aesthetic outcomes. However, one must always be conscious of publication bias in which favorable results tend to be reported and published more often. Furthermore, as hand surgeons develop innovative approaches to solve upper extremity problems, and the indications of dermal skin substitutes continue to evolve, more comparative prospective trials are needed to evaluate the long-term benefits of dermal skin substitutes in the context of reconstructive surgery.

REFERENCES

1. Halim AS, Khoo TL, Mohd Yussof SJ. Biologic and synthetic skin substitutes: an overview. Indian J Plast Surg 2010;43(Suppl):S23–8.
2. Yannas IV, Burke JF, Orgill DP, et al. Wound tissue can utilize a polymeric template to synthesize a functional extension of skin. Science 1982;215:174–6.
3. Burke JF, Yannas IV, Quinby WC Jr, et al. Successful use of a physiologically acceptable artificial skin in the treatment of extensive burn injury. Ann Surg 1981;194(4):413–28.
4. Jacoby SM, Bachoura A, Chen NC, et al. One-stage Integra coverage for fingertip injuries. Hand (N Y) 2013;8:291–5.
5. Janis JE, Kwon RK, Attinger CE. The new reconstructive ladder: modifications to the traditional

model. Plast Reconstr Surg 2011;127(Suppl 1): 205S–12S.

6. Límová M. Active wound coverings: bioengineered skin and dermal substitutes. Surg Clin North Am 2010;90(6):1237–55.

7. Shores JT, Gabriel A, Gupta S. Skin substitutes and alternatives: a review. Adv Skin Wound Care 2007; 20:493–508.

8. Lou RB, Hickerson WL. The use of skin substitutes in hand burns. Hand Clin 2009;25(4):497–509.

9. Moiemen NS, Vlachou E, Staiano JJ, et al. Reconstructive surgery with Integra dermal regeneration template: histologic study, clinical evaluation, and current practice. Plast Reconstr Surg 2006; 117(Suppl 7):160S–74S.

10. Moiemen N, Yarrow J, Hodgson E, et al. Long-term clinical and histological analysis of Integra dermal regeneration template. Plast Reconstr Surg 2011; 127(3):1149–54.

11. Iorio ML, Shuck J, Attinger CE. Wound healing in the upper and lower extremities: a systematic review on the use of acellular dermal matrices. Plast Reconstr Surg 2012;130(5 Suppl 2):232S–41S.

12. Heimbach D, Luterman A, Burke J, et al. Artificial dermis for major burns. A multi-center randomized clinical trial. Ann Surg 1988;208:313–20.

13. Shirley R, Teare L, Dziewulski P, et al. A fatal case of toxic shock syndrome associated with skin substitute. Burns 2010;36(6):e96–8.

14. Rizzo M. The use of Integra in hand and upper extremity surgery. J Hand Surg Am 2012;37(3):583–6.

15. Moiemen NS, Yarrow J, Kamel D, et al. Topical negative pressure therapy: does it accelerate neovascularisation within the dermal regeneration template, Integra? A prospective histological in vivo study. Burns 2010;36(6):764–8.

16. Bloemen MC, van der Wal MB, Verhaegen PD, et al. Clinical effectiveness of dermal substitution in burns by topical negative pressure: a multicenter randomized controlled trial. Wound Repair Regen 2012; 20(6):797–805.

17. Available at: www.fda.gov/MedicalDevices/ProductsandMedicalProcedures/DeviceApprovalsandClearances/Recently-ApprovedDevices. Accessed December 12, 2013.

18. Hop MJ, Bloemen MC, van Baar ME, et al, TOPSKIN Study Group. Cost study of dermal substitutes and topical negative pressure in the surgical treatment of burns. Burns 2013. http://dx.doi.org/10.1016/j.burns.2013.08.025. pii:S0305–4179(13)00264-7.

19. Ryssel H, Germann G, Kloeters O, et al. Dermal substitution with Matriderm® in burns on the dorsum of the hand. Burns 2010;36(8):1248–53.

20. Dantzer E, Queruel P, Salinier L, et al. Dermal regeneration template for deep hand burns: clinical utility for both early grafting and reconstructive surgery. Br J Plast Surg 2003;56(8):764–74.

21. Cuadra A, Correa G, Roa R, et al. Functional results of burned hands treated with Integra®. J Plast Reconstr Aesthet Surg 2012;65(2):228–34.

22. Haslik W, Kamolz LP, Manna F, et al. Management of full-thickness skin defects in the hand and wrist region: first long-term experiences with the dermal matrix Matriderm. J Plast Reconstr Aesthet Surg 2010;63(2):360–4.

23. Hudson DA, Renshaw A. An algorithm for the release of burn contractures of the extremities. Burns 2006;32(6):663–8.

24. Frame JD, Still J, Lakhel-LeCoadou A, et al. Use of dermal regeneration template in contracture release procedures: a multicenter evaluation. Plast Reconstr Surg 2004;113(5):1330–8.

25. Katrana F, Kostopoulos E, Delia G, et al. Reanimation of thumb extension after upper extremity degloving injury treated with Integra. J Hand Surg Eur Vol 2008;33(6):800–2.

26. Wolter TP, Noah EM, Pallua N. The use of Integra in an upper extremity avulsion injury. Br J Plast Surg 2005;58(3):416–8.

27. Graham GP, Helmer SD, Haan JM, et al. The use of Integra® Dermal Regeneration Template in the reconstruction of traumatic degloving injuries. J Burn Care Res 2013;34(2):261–6.

28. Taras JS, Sapienza A, Roach JB, et al. Acellular dermal regeneration template for soft tissue reconstruction of the digits. J Hand Surg Am 2010;35(3): 415–21.

29. Helgeson MD, Potter BK, Evans KN, et al. Bio-artificial dermal substitute: a preliminary report on its use for the management of complex combat-related soft tissue wounds. J Orthop Trauma 2007; 21(6):394–9.

30. Chalmers RL, Smock E, Geh JL. Experience of Integra(®) in cancer reconstructive surgery. J Plast Reconstr Aesthet Surg 2010;63(12):2081–90.

31. Pauchot J, Elkhyat A, Rolin G, et al. Dermal equivalents in oncology: benefit of one-stage procedure. Dermatol Surg 2013;39(1 Pt 1):43–50.

32. Smock ED, Barabas AG, Geh JL. Reconstruction of a thumb defect with Integra following wide local excision of a subungual melanoma. J Plast Reconstr Aesthet Surg 2010;63(1):e36–7.

33. Carothers JT, Brigman BE, Rizzo M. Stacking of a dermal regeneration template for reconstruction of a soft-tissue defect after tumor excision from the palm of the hand: a case report. J Hand Surg 2005;30(6):1322–6.

34. Chang SC, Miller G, Halbert CF, et al. Limiting donor site morbidity by suprafascial dissection of the radial forearm flap. Microsurgery 1996;17(3):136–40.

35. Avery CM, Pereira J, Brown AE. Suprafascial dissection of the radial forearm flap and donor site morbidity. Int J Oral Maxillofac Surg 2001;30(1): 37–41.

36. Peña I, de Villalaín L, García E, et al. Use of autologous skin equivalents with artificial dermal matrix (Integra) in donor site coverage in radial forearm free flaps: preliminary cases. J Oral Maxillofac Surg 2012;70(10):2453–8.

37. Rowe NM, Morris L, Delacure MD. Acellular dermal composite allografts for reconstruction of the radial forearm donor site. Ann Plast Surg 2006;57(3):305–11.

38. Murray RC, Gordin EA, Saigal K, et al. Reconstruction of the radial forearm free flap donor site using Integra artificial dermis. Microsurgery 2011;31(2):104–8.

39. Gravvanis AI, Tsoutsos DA, Iconomou T, et al. The use of Integra artificial dermis to minimize donor-site morbidity after suprafascial dissection of the radial forearm flap. Microsurgery 2007;27(7):583–7.

40. Medina CR, Patel SA, Ridge JA, et al. Improvement of the radial forearm flap donor defect by prelamination with human acellular dermal matrix. Plast Reconstr Surg 2011;127(5):1993–6.

41. Ellis CV, Kulber DA. Acellular dermal matrices in hand reconstruction. Plast Reconstr Surg 2012; 130(5 Suppl 2):256S–69S.

Index

Note Page numbers of article titles are in **boldface** type.

Hand Clin 30 (2014) 253–257
http://dx.doi.org/10.1016/S0749-0712(14)00015-8

hand.theclinics.com